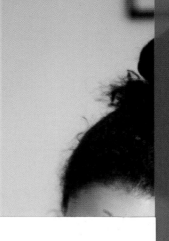

# Health Care Professionalism
## at a Glance

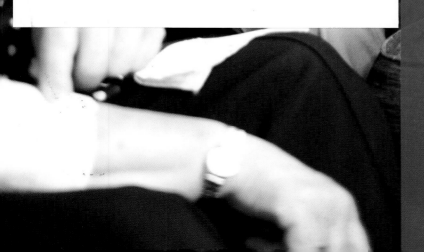

This title is also available as an e-book.
For more details, please see
**www.wiley.com/buy/9781118756386**
or scan this QR code:

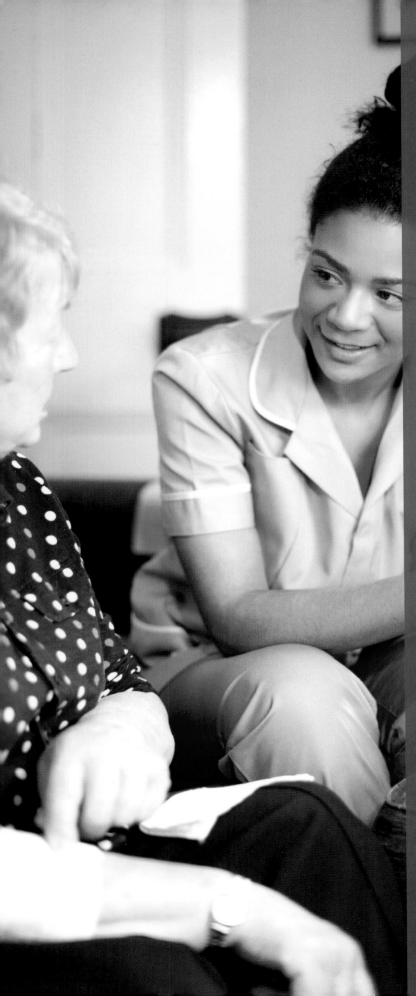

# Health Care Professionalism
# at a Glance

Edited by

**Jill Thistlethwaite**
Professor & health professions
education consultant
University of Technology Sydney
NSW Australia

**Judy McKimm**
Professor of Medical Education
College of Medicine
Swansea University
Swansea, UK

**WILEY** Blackwell

This edition first published 2016 © 2016 by John Wiley & Sons Ltd.

Registered office:     John Wiley & Sons, Ltd, The Atrium, Southern Gate, Chichester, West Sussex, PO19 8SQ, UK

Editorial offices:     9600 Garsington Road, Oxford, OX4 2DQ, UK
The Atrium, Southern Gate, Chichester, West Sussex, PO19 8SQ, UK
350 Main Street, Malden, MA 02148-5020, USA

For details of our global editorial offices, for customer services and for information about how to apply for permission to reuse the copyright material in this book please see our website at www.wiley.com/wiley-blackwell

*Library of Congress Cataloging-in-Publication Data*

Thistlethwaite, Jill, author.
   Health care professionalism at a glance / Jill Thistlethwaite, Judy McKimm.
      p. ; cm.
   Includes bibliographical references and index.
   ISBN 978-1-118-75638-6 (pbk.)
   I. McKimm, Judy, author.   II. Title.
   [DNLM:   1. Health Personnel.   2. Professional Competence.   3. Professional Practice.   W 21]
   RT82
   610.7306'9—dc23
                                                          2015000702
A catalogue record for this book is available from the British Library.

Wiley also publishes its books in a variety of electronic formats. Some content that appears in print may not be available in electronic books.

Cover image: iStock © sturti

Set in 9.5/11.5 Minion Pro Regular by Aptara Inc, New Delhi, India
Printed in Singapore

1    2015

# Contents

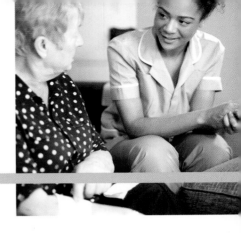

# Contributors

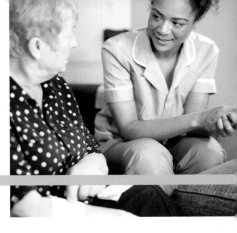

**Menna Brown**
Tutor
College of Medicine
Swansea University
Swansea, UK

**George Ridgway**
Lecturer
Learning Centre
The University of Sydney
Sydney, Australia

# Preface

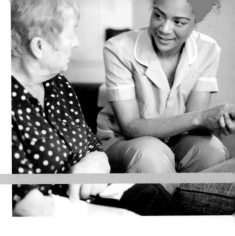

The concept of professionalism is currently the focus of much research and public interest, with an ever-increasing number of publications across many professions and disciplines. 'Professionalism' comprises a number of professional behaviours and areas for discussion and, although there is no single simple definition, it is a core requirement for all health professionals. Professional behaviours and attributes are included in curricula and competency frameworks. In this book we consider the key features of professionalism that health professional students are expected to acquire as well as how they are taught, learned and assessed. Each chapter takes one topic, introduces key definitions and explores important aspects relevant to learners and novice professionals. The chapters do not go into great detail but aim to raise questions, stimulate reflection and signpost further learning and readings. They include case scenarios, points for discussion and key references. We conclude with further reading for those of you who want to pursue topics in greater depth. As with many areas in medicine and health care, the concept of professionalism is constantly changing and so there are differences of opinion about some of the topics in the book, which help to generate stimulating conversations. Finally, although much of the text is aimed at medical students and doctors in training in the UK and western countries, the book is useful and interesting for all health professionals, including teachers and supervisors in any context. We hope you enjoy it.

*Jill Thistlethwaite*
*Judy McKimm*

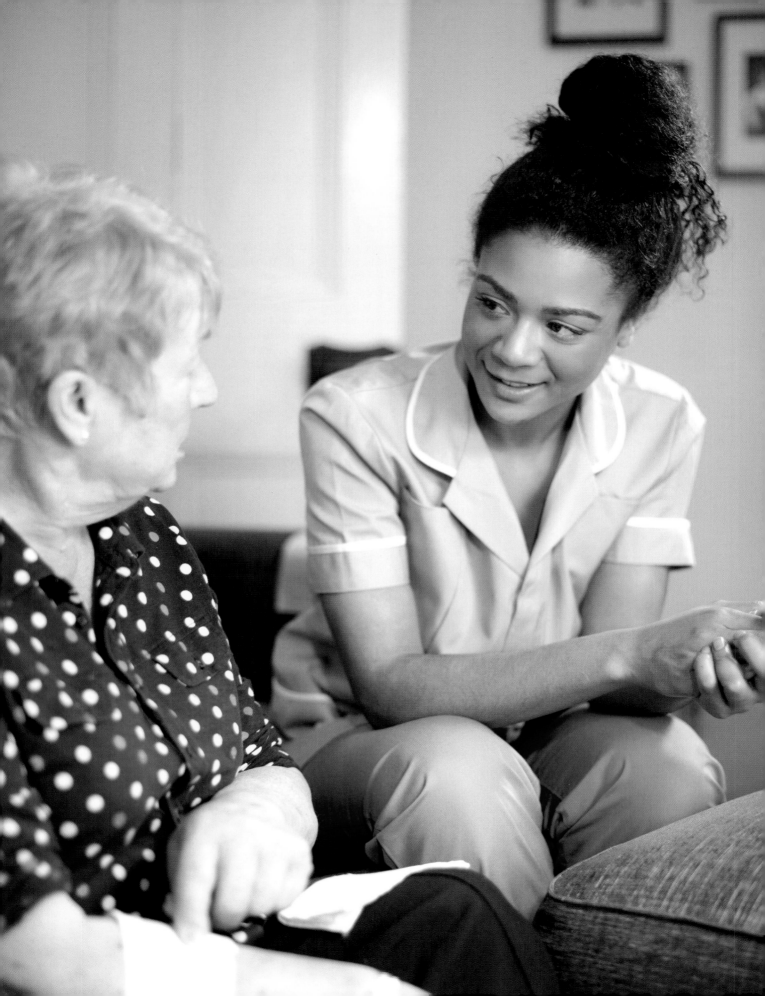

# Professionalism in context

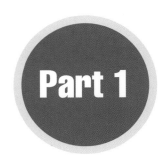

**Part 1**

## Chapters

# 1  What is professionalism?

- Definitions of a profession
- Definitions of professionalism
- Components of professionalism

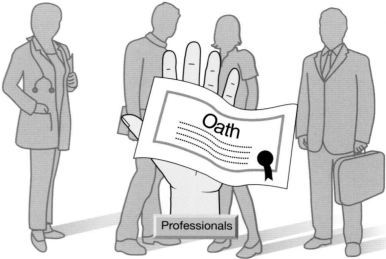

Oath

Professionals

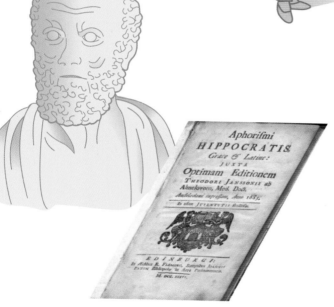

Reproduced with permission of the University of Sydney Library.

Which of the following occupations would you define as a profession and why?

- Medicine
- Nursing
- Pharmacy
- Chiropractic
- Teaching
- Politics
- Accountancy
- Law

How would you expect a professional to behave in each of the professions you have chosen?

*Health Care Professionalism at a Glance*, First Edition. Jill Thistlethwaite and Judy McKimm.
© 2016 by John Wiley & Sons, Ltd. Published 2016 by John Wiley & Sons, Ltd.

*The bond between a man and his profession is similar to that which ties him to his country; it is just as complex, often ambivalent, and in general it is understood completely only when it is broken: by exile or emigration in the case of one's country, by retirement in the case of a trade or profession. (Primo Levi, chemist and writer, in: Other People's Trades 1985, trans. 1989)*

In this introductory chapter we consider the nature of professionalism, its relationship to being a member of a profession and why all this is important for health care professionals.

# Definitions

*Professionalism: the competence or skill expected of a professional* — Oxford English Dictionary, 2nd edition, 2003.
    *'It's NOT the job you DO, It's HOW you DO the job'* –
anonymous at:
    http://clancycross.com/2009/03/26/professional-attitude/
    *A professional is a member of a profession* – derived from the Latin word *profiteri* meaning to avow or profess; for example, many doctors *profess* the Hippocratic oath when they qualify.

This all seems simple so far but the literature on professionalism, particularly in relation to medicine, has been expanding markedly in the last few decades and there is still much debate about what actually constitutes professionalism, particularly in relation to 'professional' and 'unprofessional' behaviour.

One sociologist lists the following attributes of a *profession:*
- A skill set based on specialist knowledge
- Provision of training and education
- Means of testing for competence
- Organisation of members
- Adherence to a code of conduct
- The provision of an altruistic service not just for financial reward (Johnson, 1972)

Putting this all together is the following contemporary definition from 2004:

*A profession is 'an occupation whose core element is work based upon the mastery of a complex body of knowledge and skills. It is a vocation in which knowledge of some department of science or learning or the practice of an art founded upon it is used in the service of others. Its members are governed by codes of ethics and profess a commitment to competence, integrity and morality, altruism and the promotion of the common good within their domain' (Cruess et al., 2004).*

The attributes of professionalism are also related to their being a social contract between the profession and society. This contract gives the profession a degree of autonomy and self-regulation, but in return society expects that professionals are accountable to those they serve, their profession and society (Cruess et al., 2004).

**The code of conduct** — how to behave — is the essence of professionalism (see Chapter 20). Health professional training now introduces students to the code of their specific profession, which includes ethical and legal requirements. Professionalism is taught through formal and informal activities, and students are expected to learn the correct way to behave. Moreover, professionalism and professional behaviour is now assessed through a variety of means.

A professional is
    '...a man who can do his job when he doesn't feel like it. An amateur is a man who can't do his job when he does feel like it.' James Agate (1877—1947), British diarist and critic
    'a reflective practitioner who acts ethically'. Hilton and Slotnick (2005)

Think of three examples of professional behaviour and three examples of unprofessional behaviour. How do you make the distinction based on the definitions above? Can students behave unprofessionally? Is unprofessional behaviour likely to vary for students of different professions?

# Professionalism courses

Can professionalism be taught? Well, you will certainly find teaching related to professionalism at university.

The most common components of professionalism courses, which are often called personal and professional development (PPD), are
- Ethics and the duties of a health professional
- The law applied to health professional practice
- The role of the regulatory body (e.g. for medicine — the General Medical Council in the United Kingdom and the Australian Health Professional Regulatory Authority and the medical boards in Australia; for nursing — the Nursing and Midwifery Council in the United Kingdom and the Nursing and Midwifery Board in Australia)
- Communication (not only with patients but also with colleagues/other health professionals; and not only oral but also written and online)
- Teamwork and collaboration
- Self-care
- Cultural awareness and cultural competence
- Reflective practice
- Patient safety
- Leadership

There may also be discussions about professional attributes such as altruism, empathy and compassion — raising the question of whether these can be taught and indeed learned. Some schools include teaching on professional autonomy, evidence-based practice and values-based practice under 'professionalism'.

# 2 Health professionalism

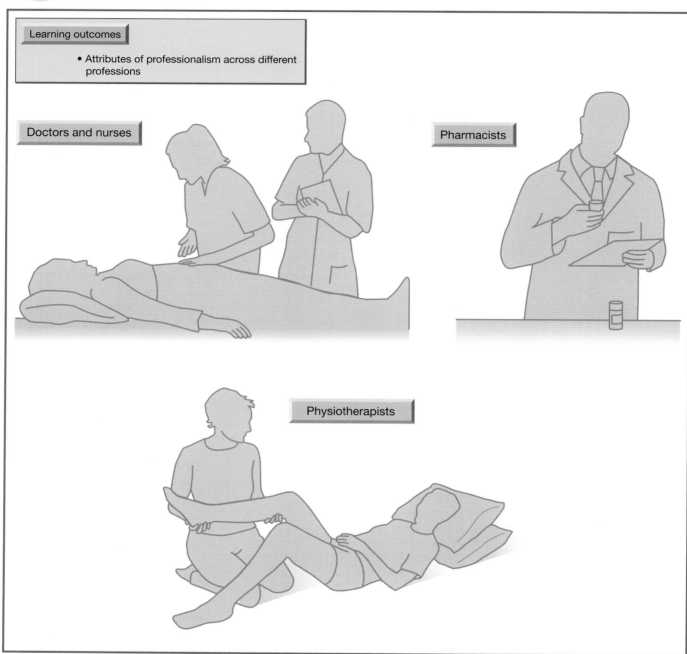

In this chapter, we provide examples of how professionalism is discussed in health professional charters and lists of competencies. A competency is an observable ability that develops through stages of expertise from novice to expert. A more recent term is **entrustable professional activity** (EPA): a key task of a profession that can be entrusted to an individual who possesses the appropriate level of competencies (Frank et al., 2010). There is not enough space to consider each health profession, but the following gives an idea of the theme and flavours of professionalism around the globe.

> Compare the items and attributes in the various lists. What are the similarities and differences, and what might account for these? Are there any that surprise you?

## Medicine

**Medical Professionalism in the New Millennium: A Physician's Charter (American Board of Internal Medicine — ABIM, 2002)**
Medical professionalism is underpinned by

**Three fundamental principles**
- Primacy of patient welfare
- Primacy of patient autonomy
- Principle of social justice

**Ten professional responsibilities**
- Professional competence
- Honesty with patients
- Patient confidentiality
- Maintaining appropriate relationships with patients
- Improving quality of care
- Improving access to care
- Just distribution of resources
- Scientific knowledge
- Maintaining trust by managing conflicts of interest
- Professional responsibilities

The General Medical Council (UK) defines three main roles for medical students:

1 The doctor as a scholar and a scientist
2 The doctor as a practitioner
3 The doctor as a **professional**

Similarly, the Australian Medical Council has four domains:
1 Science and scholarship
2 Clinical practice — doctor as a practitioner
3 Health and society — doctor as a health advocate
4 **Professionalism** and leadership

If you are a medical student, think about what each of these means and how you will develop them during your training.

## Nursing

The code of professional conduct for nurses in Australia, as defined by the Nursing and Midwifery Board (2008), includes that nurses
- Practise in a safe and competent manner
- Practise in accordance with the standards of the profession and broader health system

- Practise and conduct themselves in accordance with laws relevant to the profession and the practice of nursing
- Respect the dignity, culture, ethnicity, values and beliefs of people receiving care and treatment, and of their colleagues
- Treat personal information obtained in a professional capacity as private and confidential
- Provide impartial, honest and accurate information in relation to nursing care and health care products
- Support the health, well-being and informed decision-making of people requiring or receiving care
- Promote and preserve the trust and privilege inherent in the relationship between nurses and people receiving care
- Maintain and build on the community's trust and confidence in the nursing profession
- Practise nursing reflectively and ethically

The Best Practice Guidelines relating to professionalism in nursing from Registered Nurses' Association of Ontario, Canada (RNAO, 2007) also lists
- Being committed to lifelong learning
- Recognising personal capabilities, knowledge base and areas for development
- Working independently and exercising decision-making within one's appropriate scope of practice
- Becoming aware of barriers and constraints that may interfere with one's autonomy and seeking ways to remedy the situation
- Advocacy – being knowledgeable about policies that impact on delivery of health care

If you are a nursing student, think about what each of these means and how you will develop them during your training.

## Physiotherapy

The Chartered Society of Physiotherapy (2014) (United Kingdom) defines professionalism and its dimensions including
- Clinical reasoning and decision-making within changing, uncertain and unpredictable situations
- The requirement to work as part of a wider multi-professional team and not just in isolation
- The need to cope with the unknown and unexpected, as well as the routine

> Look up professionalism in the accreditation standards of other professions, and for your own if not mentioned here. Is anything missing that you think should be included?

## Professionalism in the 21st century

Becoming a health professional is challenging and stimulating. New challenges occur as discoveries are made, new technologies are embraced and new professions emerge. In the last decade health professionals have had to grapple with complex issues such as electronic communication with patients, social media, the mapping of the human genome and its implications, cloning, social justice and the ever increasing cost of health care. Learning never stops and competency needs to be maintained: hallmarks of being professional.

# 3  Brief history of the profession of medicine

## Definition

A 'profession' is defined by the Oxford Dictionary as being 'a paid occupation, especially one that involves prolonged training and a formal qualification'. And 'the profession' describes a body of people engaged in a particular profession; here we are talking about **doctors** engaged in **the medical profession** as an example of one of the earliest health professions to be established.

## Professions

The earliest professions were those of law, divinity and medicine. They were characterised by having a formal, university-based educational process and apprenticeship-based training; restricting entry to those who met certain criteria and controlling membership at various stages through examinations and length of service and experience. For example, in the European Union, to facilitate the free movement of doctors and equivalence of training, all medical graduates (at point of full registration) are (since October 2013) expected to have studied for 5 years and 5500 hours. This places constraints on the programmes universities and schools provide, and (without a definition of common learning outcomes or assessment) does not guarantee that all doctors qualifying in the EU countries will be of a similar standard. Postgraduate training in most countries specifies the examinations to be taken and passed before a doctor can take on a particular role as well as length of time to be served at each level.

The existence of professions brings many benefits to individuals (e.g. work autonomy, high status, financial reward) and to society (e.g. through improving health or education or maintaining justice). However, some sociologists (e.g. Foucault, Freidson, see *Further Reading*) have criticised the establishment of professions in perpetuating restrictive, elitist and monopoly-based practices and maintaining occupational closure. Such writers emphasise the way in which professions create, use and hold onto power to control members of the profession, to place boundaries around a body of knowledge and expertise and to maintain prestige and authority within society.

What mechanisms does the medical profession use to create use and hold onto power? How do you think these have changed in the last two decades and why?

## Medicine

Before the 1800s, much dentistry and minor surgery was carried out by barbers who were cheaper than doctors, easier to access and had good knife skills. A deeper understanding of human anatomy and technical and pharmaceutical advances led to doctors being able to diagnose diseases more accurately and perform more advanced surgical techniques. Subsequently, physicians and surgeons (and apothecaries) became defined as part of the medical profession and their activities were defined and regulated by law. Now anyone who is not licensed cannot perform such activities unless they are granted a special licence.

Professions are regulated by formal, statutory bodies and doctors as individuals are licensed and regulated by medical councils or boards. Education and training is also regulated by councils, and the organisations who are accredited to provide medical education and training are usually listed in a Medical Act (or equivalent). Doctors' professional powers and rights to practise are also enshrined in legislation, professional standards, guidance and an ethical code of conduct.

Of course, medicine itself is constantly changing as the profession responds to societal change and expectations, which will vary from culture to culture and over time. There has been a shift in many Western countries over the last few decades from a more paternalistic and sometimes patronising approach in which what the doctor said was unquestioned, to a policy rhetoric and practice which uses very different language: for example 'patient partnership', the 'expert patient' and 'empowerment'. Similarly, doctors and the profession itself are now much more accountable to the public in the wake of scandals and failures which highlighted the need for more objective and robust regulation than that which had traditionally been carried out by the profession itself.

### The professional in practice

What patients want from their doctors is not only to be well-cared for clinically, but also to be communicated with clearly and appropriately. For many years, students and doctors have learned and been assessed on their communication skills; the way in which medical information is now freely available on the Internet is starting to change the way in which doctors 'control' information. How might you, as an individual practitioner, ensure that whilst you retain your identity as a professional with expertise and knowledge, you also facilitate empowering patients? Although this may feel like losing or giving away power, you are actually helping patients and families take responsibility and care for themselves – this is empowerment. We explore these issues further in later chapters.

## Changing professional roles

The nature and activities of different professions are constantly changing and being redefined in the light of societal, economic and political changes. Now, many professions exist, although there is some variance between countries and cultures. In health care, we have seen a movement towards extending the scope of practice of traditional professions (e.g. prescribing pharmacists, midwives and advanced practitioners) as well as the creation of new professionals, such as physician assistants.

> List all the health professions you can think of. Do you think all of them fit the definitions of 'profession' described above? What difficulties might you (or have you) encountered as health professionals extend or expand their scope of practice into areas which have traditionally been those of doctors?

Finally, the widespread use of social media also impacts on how colleagues and patients might view doctors and how professional identity is seen which is explored further in Chapter 8.

# Becoming a professional

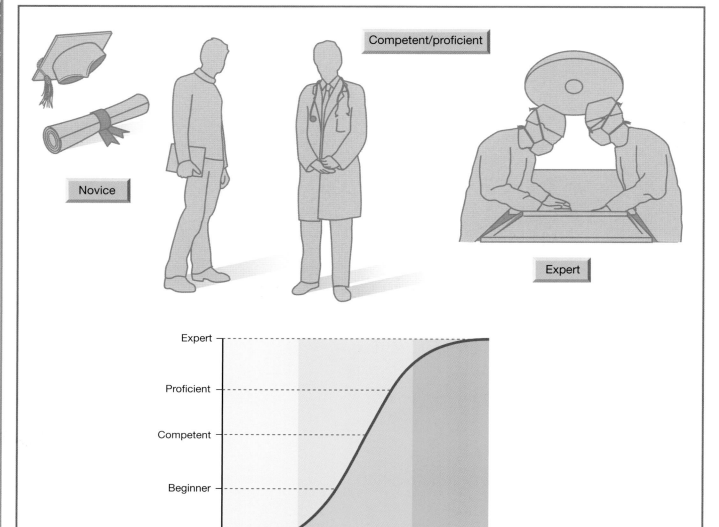

The Dreyfus and Dreyfus 'Novice to Expert' model

## LPP

**L**egitimate–a status is conferred on the 'novice'–they are legitimately allowed to be part of the community

**P**eripheral–they start on the edge, and gradually work their way into the community through the 'inbound trajectory'

**P**articipation–they are required and encouraged to participate, they become part of the community by participating

*Health Care Professionalism at a Glance*, First Edition. Jill Thistlethwaite and Judy McKimm.
© 2016 by John Wiley & Sons, Ltd. Published 2016 by John Wiley & Sons, Ltd.

The process of becoming and being a professional is not one that is ever completed, but is a continuing, lifelong journey. Informal and work-based learning, role modelling and the hidden curriculum interact and work alongside the formal curriculum to educate, inform and develop individual professional identities. Aspiring health professionals must navigate the intricacies of each to understand how the actions of others impact upon their own professionalism and acknowledge and reflect upon their own actions and behaviours, which in turn shape the professional identity of others. We can consider this process from a number of perspectives.

## Socialisation

One way of describing the process of becoming a professional is to think of it as being socialised ('enculturated' or 'acculturated') into not only your own specific health profession but also into the way in which health care is viewed and delivered. This varies over time between cultures and professions and explains how professional identity is acquired through learning the language, norms, values, rituals, behaviours and social skills relevant to the social position. Becker and colleagues' classic book, *Boys in White* (Becker et al., 1961), described the experience of primarily middle class, male medical students at an US school. Contrast this with Sinclair's *Making Doctors* about a UK medical school (Sinclair, 1997) and you can see that, whereas some of the rituals, behaviours and values remain, there have been huge changes over time and between cultures. Once an individual has acquired and/or learned to display the relevant norms, values, and so on, then they become an accepted member of that culture and can perform the required activities and role appropriately. They are also aware of the boundaries between themselves, other professionals, patients and families.

> Can you think of some examples of language, norms, values and rituals that would be unacceptable now, but were commonplace decades ago? And vice versa?
> What are some of the ways in which health professionals are socialised into their profession and health services?

## Rites of passage

One of the ways in which students and graduates are socialised into universities and into their professions is through 'rites of passage'. Rites of passage usually involve some initiation ceremony, mark a transition from one stage of life to another and typically confer new responsibilities. They include rituals such as 'freshers' week' for new students; graduation ceremonies; reading of oaths or other agreements; and employment induction courses. These rites of passage often involve a change in clothing or title (e.g. wearing of a uniform, white coat, stethoscope or being given a professional title).

## Tribes and territories

Another way of thinking about the different subcultures that inhabit health care and universities is in terms of 'tribes and territories' (Becher and Trowler, 2001).

> List some of the tribes and territories found in hospitals, in primary care and in social services.
> What are the key features and behaviours of some of these 'tribes'?
> What is helpful, and what is unhelpful about belonging or not belonging to these tribes?

Medical specialties, different health and social care professions and academic disciplines all have distinguishing features and ways of 'being and behaving'. Belonging to a tribe can feel very comforting: it is good to know that you belong, that you are an anatomist, a surgeon, a nurse, a physiotherapist or a paramedic. And when belonging comes with a territory, which may be physical space (e.g. a dissection room, an operating theatre or an ambulance), or a body of knowledge, equipment or control over time, then this can give some tribes more power or status than others and even lead to 'tribal warfare'. Such 'warfare' may be characterised by miscommunication, or conflict between professions and specialties, which ultimately may adversely affect the care of patients.

## Communities of practice

Part of becoming professionalised is to acquire the skills and competencies that the profession requires. Benner (1984) builds on earlier work in considering how professionals become 'expert', as they move through stages from novice, advanced beginner, competent, proficient, expertise to mastery (the expert level). This can refer to simple skill sets (e.g. aseptic technique) or to 'an expert' who has mastery over many aspects of their work. Experts typically take some risks (they will try new things) and use deliberate practice as a way of becoming expert. If, as research has shown, chess masters or concert pianists need 10,000 hours of practice to become expert, then it is no surprise that the road to becoming an expert health professional is equally long.

Lave and Wenger (1991) provide another way of conceptualising this development towards being 'expert' in their description of 'communities of practice'. Newcomers to the 'community' (e.g. student midwives or physiotherapists) engage in 'legitimate peripheral participation' (LPP) and, by so doing, become part of that community and eventually become expert through mastery. Another helpful concept, that of 'entrustable professional activities' (ten Cate, 2013) describes a framework whereby learners are trusted by both their trainers and patients to engage in gradually more difficult activities through an increasing demonstration of their expertise.

# 5 Role of regulatory and professional bodies

**Learning outcomes:**

- The role of regulatory and professional bodies
- Standards, competencies and outcomes
- Registration
- Codes of practice

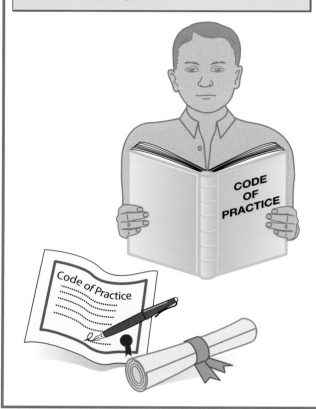

**UK Health and Care Professions' Council standards of conduct, performance and ethics**

1 You must act in the best interest of service users.
2 You must respect the confidentiality of service users.
3 You must keep high standards of personal conduct.
4 You must provide (to us and any other relevant regulators) any important information about your conduct and competence.
5 You must keep your professional knowledge and skills up to date.
6 You must act within the limits of your knowledge, skills and experience and, if necessary, refer the matter to another practitioner.
7 You must communicate properly and effectively with service users and other practitioners.
8 You must effectively supervise tasks that you have asked other people to carry out.
9 You must get informed consent to provide care or services (so far as possible).
10 You must keep accurate records.
11 You must deal fairly and safely with the risks of infection.
12 You must limit your work or stop practising if your performance or judgement is affected by your health.
13 You must behave with honesty and integrity and make sure that your behaviour does not damage the public's confidence in you or your profession.
14 You must make sure that any advertising you do is accurate.

www.hcpc-uk.org/assets/documents/10003B6EStandardssofconduct,performanceandethics.pdf

*Health Care Professionalism at a Glance*, First Edition. Jill Thistlethwaite and Judy McKimm.
© 2016 by John Wiley & Sons, Ltd. Published 2016 by John Wiley & Sons, Ltd.

Some of the key aspects that make an occupation 'professional' is that its body of knowledge is codified and defined, and entrance to the profession is controlled by a formal gatekeeping process, which includes the broader defining of skills and professional attributes or qualities.

## Regulatory, statutory and professional bodies

In line with the above description, in order to protect the public and ensure that only those who are suitably qualified can practise that profession, a number of formal bodies and organisations have been established. Although these vary from country to country (including the establishment of regional bodies), some general principles apply.

Most professions are regulated by a body which is given statutory powers by government or the state. These are typically known as 'Councils', 'Agencies' or 'Colleges', e.g. the UK Health and Care Professions' Council; the Australian Health Practitioner Regulation Agency or the Health Regulatory Colleges in Canada. Such bodies grant a licence to practise and hold the register of practising professionals and, either alone, or in collaboration with other bodies, set the standards or competencies which a member of that profession must meet and maintain. In many countries, a federation or overarching council exists which brings together a range of bodies regulating individual health professions. This helps ensure more consistency across and between professions, and can be particularly helpful when new professions are being established or in cases of major review.

Other types of professional associations have a more indirect role in maintaining professionalism. These include educational organisations which produce best practice curriculum guidance (e.g. the Institute of Medical Ethics), bodies such as the Medical Royal Colleges that define postgraduate curricula in every medical specialty, and professional associations (or 'unions') that assist their members through providing advice, insurance and guidance on a range of professional issues. Many of these organisations, as do regulatory bodies, also carry out research into and consultations on broader topical issues to advise the profession or government.

> What are the main regulatory and professional bodies that govern your profession? Are you aware of all the guidance and activities that they provide or undertake?

## Standards and competencies

Every regulated profession has its own set of professional standards which have been developed through consultation with key stakeholders and reference to international examples. Although the language might vary between professions and over time, most guidance documents are set out in terms of either core standards, competencies or outcomes at various levels which correspond to points of registration.

Such guidance is typically defined under specific headings relating to

- Underpinning knowledge and understanding
- Practical, clinical or procedural skills or competencies
- Professional attributes or behaviours (including communication, team-working and leadership)
- Commitment to continuing professional development

In order to ensure a consistent high standard of entry-level professionals, most professions are now moving towards requiring an undergraduate (bachelors) degree for initial registration and licensing. In some professions and countries, achievement of the degree is sufficient for entry to the register. In others, an additional examination, extra evidence or an additional 'internship' or further training period is required before a full licence for independent practice is granted. Such requirements provide the main means of controlling entry to the profession.

> How are the standards or competencies for entry to your profession defined? Take a look at either a set of standards for your profession from another country or those of another profession and compare the similarities and differences.

Beyond initial entry to the register, regulatory bodies are usually responsible for maintaining the register of practising professionals. In some professions, different sections of the register apply to professionals with additional post-qualifying qualifications or experience (e.g. postgraduate degrees or specialisms; advanced practice qualifications which extend their scope of practice) or for professionals with a limited scope of practice. Increasingly, professionals are required to carry out regular, ongoing activities to demonstrate their continuing professional development and remain on the register (see Chapter 7). International professionals are usually required to undertake entrance examinations or provide a range of evidence prior to being awarded a licence to practise although some countries/professions have reciprocal agreements.

## Codes of practice

In addition to defining the standards that individual practitioners have to achieve, regulatory and professional bodies also set out professional codes of practice to which all their professionals have to adhere. These codes are usually set out in terms of an ethical and legal framework; professional conduct and behaviours and standards of performance. Adherence to these codes of practice is fundamental to being a professional. Underpinning the code of practice is the concept of 'Fitness to Practise' which includes displaying the appropriate professional behaviours and being physically and psychologically fit to practise the profession without putting patients, colleagues or yourself at risk (see Chapter 6).

# 6 Fitness to practise and health for practice

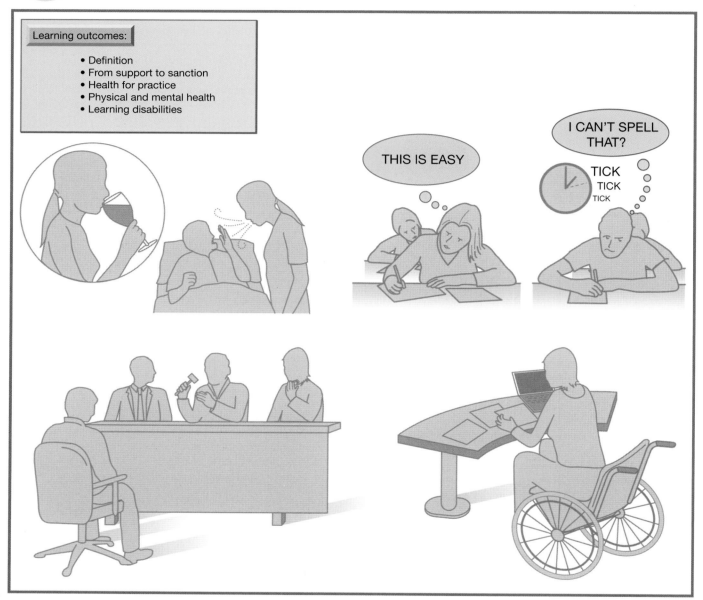

Learning outcomes:
- Definition
- From support to sanction
- Health for practice
- Physical and mental health
- Learning disabilities

THIS IS EASY

I CAN'T SPELL THAT?

TICK
TICK
TICK

## Definition

When we talk about 'fitness to practise' we mean that the individual professional (or student) has the knowledge, skills, capabilities and attributes to practise competently, ethically, legally and safely for their stage of practice in accordance with a formally defined code of conduct. Being unfit to practise may arise from acts by a student or fully licensed practitioner which may affect public protection or confidence in the profession. This may include matters not directly related to professional practice, e.g. criminal acts or public activities.

## Professional behaviours and conduct

All professions, including health professions, clearly describe and set out guidance about the behaviours and conduct expected from any member of that profession. Practitioners must be able to practise safely at every stage of education, training or practice. In some countries (e.g. Canada), students are required to join a professional register, but in the main, becoming registered occurs on graduation or shortly thereafter and is concurrent with being awarded a full licence to practise.

*Health Care Professionalism at a Glance*, First Edition. Jill Thistlethwaite and Judy McKimm.
© 2016 by John Wiley & Sons, Ltd. Published 2016 by John Wiley & Sons, Ltd.

Throughout this book, we set out various aspects of professional and unprofessional behaviours, including when and why complaints may be made about health professionals and how this relates to fitness to practise (see Chapter 37). Here we focus on issues relating to health and welfare.

## Support and sanction

Whilst many individuals may remediate unprofessional behaviours or can practice safely with a range of conditions described, in some cases this is not possible. Some behaviours (such as theft, assault, cheating, drug dealing or abuse) are incompatible with public expectations of the health professions. For some learners or practitioners, their physical or mental health conditions may require occupational health assessment and support. This will vary greatly with individual circumstances. Support may involve modifications to the learning environment or workplace, suspending studies or taking an employment break or (in some cases) ceasing study or work.

For both behavioural and serious health issues, students will typically be referred through formal departmental and university fitness to practise processes and information may be passed onto employers or bodies responsible for further training. This route is different from the academic processes that determine clinical competence and understanding (see Chapter 12). Formal assessment of professional behaviours is now seen as an increasing part of competence and learners can fail such assessments. Sanctions for student fitness to practise issues can range from an informal warning (for something deemed to be a mistake or behaviour unlikely to be repeated) to expulsion from a programme. Universities may have separate disciplinary codes and processes that all students have to abide by (e.g. plagiarism or alcohol misuse on university premises).

Registered practitioners must adhere to their profession's codes of conduct and, depending on the severity and nature of the unprofessional behaviour or condition's impact on practice, may be subject to formal fitness to practise processes. The outcome will vary depending on the context: ranging from the case being dismissed, having a reduced or limited scope of practice, or being excluded from the register and thus unable to practise.

## Health for practice

Health professionals have demanding jobs which require robust physical and psychological health. Whilst many conditions are compatible with a successful career in the health professions, conditions can become more severe, new conditions can emerge and injury or accident can lead to temporary or permanently impaired health (Dyrbye et al., 2010). Health professionals at all stages of education or employment (including pre-enrolment and pre-employment) are required to declare any conditions that may require support, occupational health assessment or affect their practice or learning (see Chapter 18 on self-care).

Physical and psychological conditions may also be disabilities. Disability is usually defined under legislation which sets out an individual's rights. In the United Kingdom, a person is disabled under the Equality Act 2010 if he/she has a physical or mental impairment that has a 'substantial' and 'long-term' negative effect on the ability to do normal daily activities (www.gov.uk/definition-of-disability-under-equality-act-2010). Long term is 12 months or more; substantial is more than minor or trivial. Employers or educational institutions are required to provide 'reasonable adjustments' under the Act.

## Physical health

Physical health includes temporary or long-term easily observed conditions (e.g. being a wheelchair user) and 'invisible' conditions such as diabetes, asthma and sensory impairments, e.g. hearing or sight impairments. It also includes infections which may put others at risk, e.g. influenza and tuberculosis. Although blood-borne viruses (e.g. HIV, hepatitis) might not preclude practising as a health professional, the scope of practice will be limited.

## Mental health

Many people will have a mental health condition at some time in their lives and health professionals are no exception. The stress of university, training and the emotional toll of caring for people in difficult circumstances can exacerbate existing conditions or lead to a new one emerging. Long-term mental health conditions may become classified as a disability.

## Learning disabilities

Common learning disabilities include dyslexia and dyspraxia, both of which can require additional support during study and employment (RCP, 2011). People with learning disabilities are (in many countries) entitled to reasonable adjustments which may include having extra time in written assessments, a note taker or voice-activated software.

The UK GMC notes that 'in most cases, health conditions and disabilities will not raise fitness to practise concerns, provided the student receives the appropriate care and reasonable adjustments necessary to study and work safely in a clinical environment' (GMC, 2009a) and this premise is echoed across the professions. In fact, not declaring or seeking the appropriate support for a condition shows a lack of insight about the possible impact on practice and would in itself raise concerns about an individual's fitness to practise. Professional bodies, employers and educational organisations stress the importance to seek help early and engage in any remediation or treatment offered (Vogan et al., 2014).

**Revalidation and remediation**

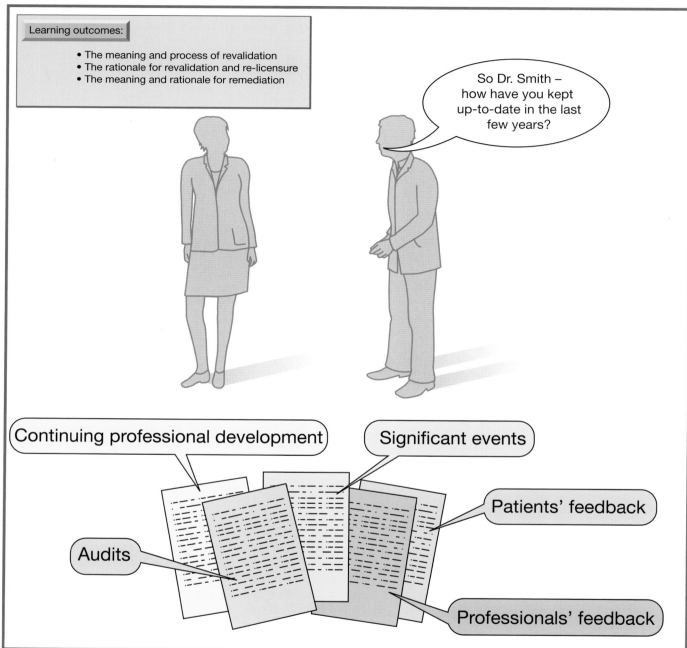

# Becoming a doctor

When you become a medical doctor you receive a license to practise from your national registration body. This is frequently the same body that provides accreditation of the institution and programme that awards the relevant medical degree (e.g. MBBS, MBChB and MD). In the United Kingdom, this is the GMC (General Medical Council). In Australia, the Medical Board through AHPRA (the Australian Health Professional Regulatory Authority) registers doctors and has given the mandate for accreditation to the AMC (Australian Medical Council). At present, in the United Kingdom and Australia there is no one national examination to become a doctor; each medical school develops and delivers its own assessment, which is vetted by the accreditation body for fitness of purpose. In Canada and the United States there is a national examination. The American version is the USMLE (United States Medical Licensing Examination) administered in three steps by the NBME (National Board of Medical Examiners).

The United Kingdom and Australia have a pre-registration year before full licensure (foundation year 1 [F1] and postgraduate year 1 [PGY1], respectively). The majority of doctors in most countries then undertake specialty training for a number of years including postgraduate examinations by the relevant bodies (e.g. the royal colleges in the United Kingdom). After this doctors are expected to remain fit to practise and to keep up-to-date as lifelong learners through continuing professional development (CPD). In many countries they have to provide evidence of attending CPD courses to retain their license or postgraduate specialisation.

# Revalidation

'The purpose of revalidation is to assure patients and the public, employers and other health care professionals that licensed doctors are up to date and fit to practise.' (GMC, 2010)

Until 1999 British doctors were able to work in their profession for life unless removed from the GMC register for unprofessional behaviour, including criminal misconduct, following a complaint. In 2002, after a series of high-profile incidents (including the Bristol Royal Infirmary paediatric surgery scandal), and public inquiries relating to patient safety, the GMC mandated that all doctors should undergo regular review of performance. This process of annual review is called 'revalidation' (synonymous with re-licensure). The introduction of revalidation was delayed for some years in part due to the case of GP Harold Shipman, who was found guilty of murdering 15 patients with intravenous opiates (though he probably likely killed more than 300 in 24 years). The public inquiry concluded that more stringent and robust procedures were required than those suggested by the GMC including increased monitoring of GPs and their prescribing, and changes to the processes for death certification.

Mandatory revalidation was introduced in the United Kingdom in 2012 and has a number of components, which vary between specialties. The process takes place on a 5-year cycle and includes an annual appraisal and evidence of taking part in CPD. CPD activities are measured in learning credits: one credit per hour of education plus an additional one credit for proof of application of learning, that is if the doctor has made changes to his/her practice as a result of the education. Overall doctors are revalidated against the principles of *Good Medical Practice* (GMC, 2013b) and have to provide supporting evidence to show they have met those principles.

## Supporting information for revalidation

The information comes under four main headings with six main types of supporting documentation required (GMC, 2012). Look at the list and consider what sort of evidence you may need under each heading and what you are collecting now as a student, in a portfolio or similar. Which areas are related to professionalism?

- General information — providing context about what you do in all aspects of your work
- Keeping up to date — maintaining and enhancing the quality of your professional work (1. CPD)
- Review of your practice — evaluating the quality of your professional work (2. Quality improvement activity; 3. Significant events)
- Feedback on your practice — how others perceive the quality of your professional work (4. Feedback from colleagues; 5. Feedback from patients; 6. Review of complaints and compliments).

# Maintenance of licensure (MoL)

In other countries revalidation is called re-licensure or recertification and varies in requirements. As there are likely to be many changes in the next five years to these processes, it is important for students and doctors to be aware of their accreditation bodies' requirements and plan accordingly. It is important to note that MoL has generated much debate about how useful it is/might be in improving doctors' practice over time, enhancing patient safety and picking up the poorly performing professionals. A criticism levelled at the UK process is that it would not identify another Harold Shipman. It is also a costly procedure. There does need to be research into the costs and the benefits as more countries adopt MoL initiatives (Boulet and van Zanten, 2014).

# Remediation

Doctors, and indeed medical students, who have problems in their performance and clinical practice, are referred for remediation.

**Remediation**: the act of correcting, putting right, reforming

Training a doctor is an expensive process — for both the individual and the state (if there is public funding involved). Therefore rather than de-register a doctor or 'expel' a poorly performing student, some form of remediation process is put into effect. This involves periods of practising under supervision, regular assessment with feedback and monitoring of patient care. However if remediation does not improve practice, in the interests of patients and the public, failing doctors and students need to be told they are unable to practise medicine.

# 8 Social media and the professional

## Menna Brown

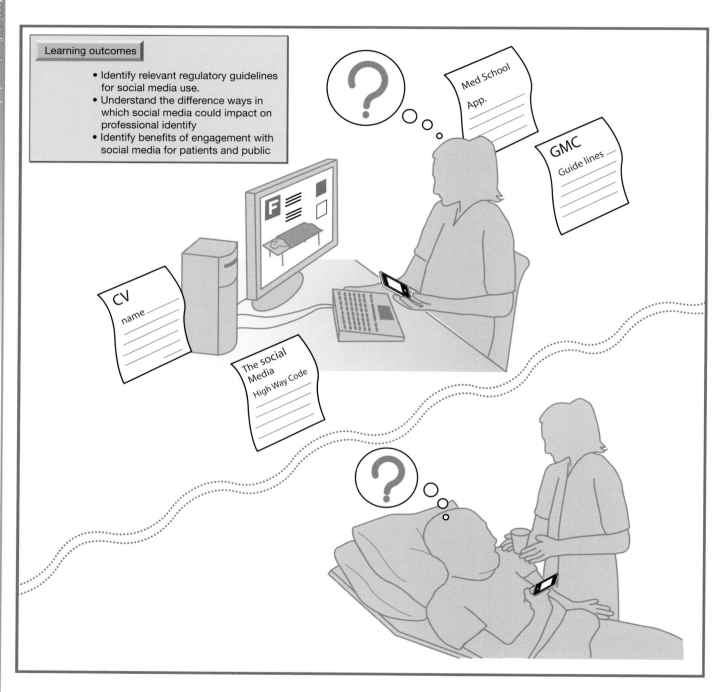

Learning outcomes

- Identify relevant regulatory guidelines for social media use.
- Understand the difference ways in which social media could impact on professional identify
- Identify benefits of engagement with social media for patients and public

*Health Care Professionalism at a Glance*, First Edition. Jill Thistlethwaite and Judy McKimm.
© 2016 by John Wiley & Sons, Ltd. Published 2016 by John Wiley & Sons, Ltd.

# Definition

'Websites and applications that enable users to create and share content or to participate in social networking' (www.oxforddictionaries.com).

Increasing use of a range of social media tools and sites has altered the way in which professionals communicate with patients and the public. These include social networking sites; Facebook, Twitter and YouTube; patient support networks; weblogs; video chat and instant messaging platforms. New technologies have required all aspiring and qualified health professionals to consider the professional image and identity they portray online. One's 'digital footprint' is a permanent record of professional behaviour and can impact on how professions are viewed collectively and by the media.

# Key regulatory policies and guidelines

Regulatory and professional bodies across all health professions are aware of the increasing influence of social media and its potential impact upon their profession and public perception. Recent publications by regulatory bodies have addressed concerns through statements and professional guidelines, for example:
- General Medical Council: Social Media Guidance (2013)
- The Royal College of Physicians. The Social Media Highway Code (2013)
- American Society of Health-System Pharmacists (ASHP) statement on use of social media by pharmacy professionals (2012)
- General Dentists Council, Social Media Guidance for Dentists (2013)
- APA Social Media Policy (2010)
- The Nursing & Midwifery Board of Australia: Information sheet on social media (2010).
- Social Media and the Medical Profession: a guide to online professionalism for medical practitioners and medical students. Joint statement by AMA, NZMA, NZMSA and AMSA (2010)

In the United Kingdom, specific regulations and guidance are provided by the Ministry of Defence for health professionals working in secured environments including the armed forces, prisons and psychiatric units.

# Risks and benefits of social media use

Numerous risks and benefits are associated with engaging and using social media for health professionals who are required to maintain a professional image. This list is not exhaustive.

## Benefits
- Improved communication and interaction with patients
- Increased access to health information and shared experiences through patient forums
- Reach wide, diverse new audiences to advertise services
- Opportunity to counteract incorrect medical information posted online to aid patient care and knowledge
- Professional networking opportunities
- Disseminate information to hard-to-reach groups

> Patient care blogs offer patients and their families the opportunity to share health experiences, exchange information and offer support to others. What resources have/could you share with your patients? How could you guide them to safe applications and reputable resources?

## Risks
- Breach patient confidentiality
- Cross professional boundaries
- Online activity may be interpreted by others as unprofessional, inappropriate, offensive, defamatory or libellous
- Posts and images are public information and a permanent record which may be accessed by patients, colleagues, peers, employers or the public at any time
- Actions may be reported to the media, employers or regulatory bodies.
- Unintended consequences of actions and behaviour online

> Julia participated in the 'lying down game' whilst on shift working as a junior doctor. She and two of her colleagues took photographs of themselves lying face down on hospital trolleys, the ward floor and helipad. The photographs were posted on Facebook and hospital management identified the hospital and staff members involved. What would you consider an appropriate response from management? How might your employer respond? Or your patients?

## The generation gap

Digital natives are considered to be those born after 1980, brought up using digital technologies. They are differentiated from those born into an analogue culture who have subsequently immigrated over. There is a generation gap between users of social media. Digital natives are often high users, widely engaged and active participants in online communities (Morris and McKimm, 2009). Regardless of generation, all health care professionals have a responsibility to update, learn or improve digital skills. Those less familiar may have a responsibility to update skills and knowledge to ensure they do not put themselves or others at risk through online interactions, while younger generations may need to consider the way in which they engage with social media and reflect on new professional identities and make appropriate changes.

> Social media impacts on how the public and patients view doctors: how might this impact on your profession or your professional identity? What does your online profile say about you? Would you be happy for a patient to view it?

As new technologies advance and develop they continue to alter the way in which health care is delivered, received and experienced by patients and the public. As a result professionals have a responsibility to consider their practices and establish safe ways of working which do not put themselves or others at risk.

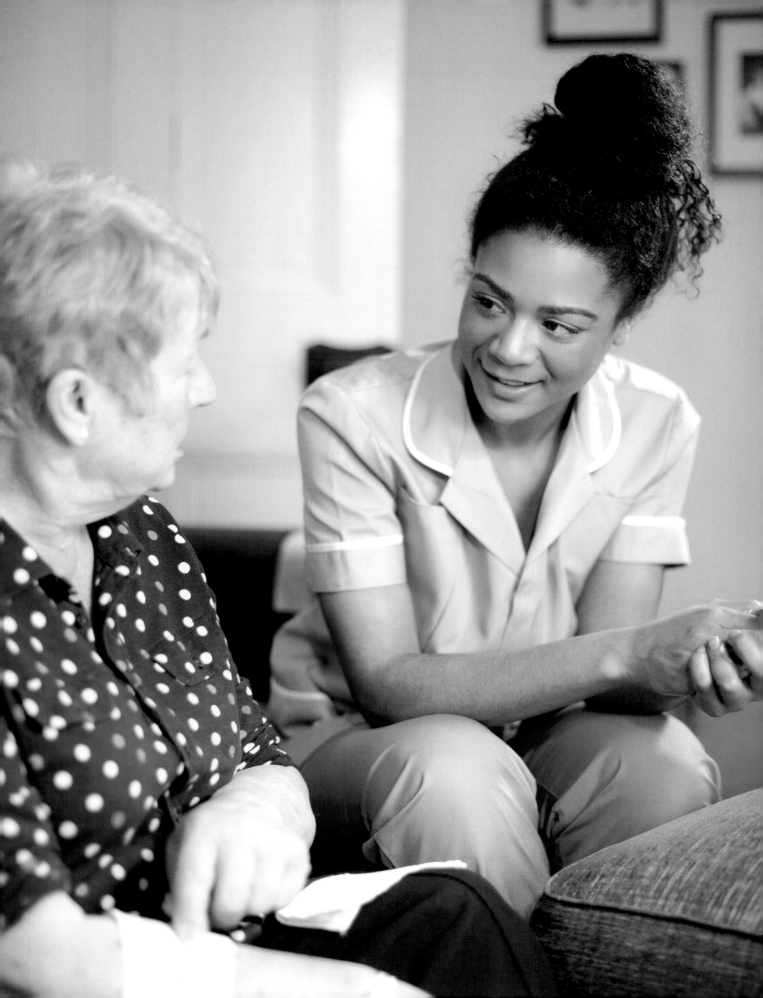

# Learning to be a professional

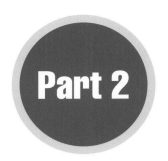

**Part 2**

## Chapters

# 9 The formal curriculum

- Definition of the formal curriculum
- Learning outcomes in relation to professionalism
- Principles in 'Good Medical Practice'
- Key aims of professional development

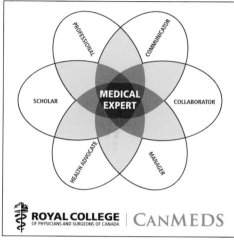

Copyright © 2005 The Royal College of Physicians and Surgeons of Canada. http://rcpsc.medical.org/canmeds. Reproduced with permission.

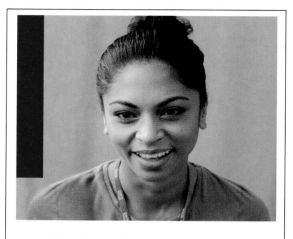

Good medical practice

General Medical Council

Regulating doctors
Ensuring good medical practice

Reproduced with permission of the General Medical Council.

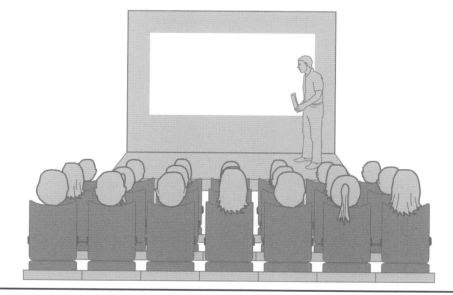

*Health Care Professionalism at a Glance*, First Edition. Jill Thistlethwaite and Judy McKimm.
© 2016 by John Wiley & Sons, Ltd. Published 2016 by John Wiley & Sons, Ltd.

# How do we learn to be professional?

*Some [college] values are caught and not taught.*
R.B. House (1948)

The above saying reflects a common assumption that professional behaviour is learnt through observation from other professionals acting as role models, if a person does not already have the requisite attributes and values when starting medical school.

> Reflect for a moment on your own behaviour. When, where and how did you 'learn' about the way you should behave in public? Is there a difference between your behaviour at school, in social situations, at medical school and in clinical settings? Who has been most influential as a role model in terms of your professional behaviour?

However, medical schools can no longer rely on learning by observation and are mandated by their national accreditation body to provide teaching and assessment of professionalism. The admission process for your university may have included methods such as interviews to assess your existing professional values and outlook but further learning is necessary to become a 'professional' doctor. And entry to postgraduate training increasingly includes assessments of professional behaviours.

## The formal curriculum – learning outcomes

At undergraduate level, the formal curriculum is a medical school's written statement of the learning outcomes it expects its graduating doctors to have achieved by the end of their programme. This curriculum should also include the activities that students will undertake to meet these outcomes and how they will be assessed. The term 'core curriculum' is also used to indicate those outcomes that **all** students must achieve. Optional activities, such as student-selected courses or special study modules, will have additional outcomes that vary depending on the topic.

Postgraduate training curricula also include learning outcomes or competences relating to professional behaviour e.g. showing respect for patients; communicating clearly and demonstrating appropriate leadership.

In this chapter we consider how core outcomes are defined and, in later chapters, the learning activities and assessments aligned with these.

The organisations that accredit medical schools so that their medical programmes are formally able to graduate doctors have more recently stipulated that professionalism must be included in the core curriculum, along with medical knowledge and clinical skills. This reflects the increasing emphasis on professional attributes and behaviours that are set out for doctors at all stages of training and practice. In the United Kingdom, the General Medical Council's guidance was first published in *Tomorrow's Doctors* in 1993. Later in the updated version, the GMC (2009) stated that *'The principles of professional practice set out in Good Medical Practice must form the basis of medical education'* and a set of learning outcomes based on these principles was defined.

- Do you know what your own school's learning outcomes are in relation to professionalism?
- You may want to compare these with those in the boxes and think about the learning and teaching necessary for you to attain them.
- Which outcomes do you feel you have already achieved?
- How would you provide evidence of this achievement?

> **Principles and issues covered in *Good Medical Practice, 2013***
> *Knowledge, skills and performance*
> - Develop and maintain your professional performance
> - Apply knowledge and experience to practice
> - Record your work clearly, accurately and legibly
>
> *Safety and quality*
> - Contribute to and comply with systems to protect patients
> - Respond to risks to safety
> - Protect patients and colleagues from any risk posed by your health (self-care)
>
> *Communication, partnership and teamwork*
> - Communicate effectively
> - Work collaboratively with colleagues to maintain or improve patient care
> - Teaching, training, supporting and assessing
> - Continuity and coordination of care
> - Establish and maintain partnerships with patients
>
> *Maintaining trust*
> - Show respect for patients
> - Treat patients and colleagues fairly and without discrimination
> - Act with honesty and integrity

These GMC-derived outcomes may be summarised as key aims.

> **Key aims of professional development during medical school**
> - To enable students to understand the origins of professionalism and the proper set of responsibilities of the profession
> - To instil and nurture in students the development of personal qualities, values, attitudes and behaviours that are fundamental to the practice of medicine and health care
> - To ensure that students understand the importance and relevance of these concepts, demonstrate these qualities at a basic level in their work and are willing to continue to develop their professional identity

The GMC has also published guidance for medical students on professional values and fitness to practise which include principles relating to good clinical care, maintaining good medical practice, teaching and training, relationships with patients, working with colleagues, probity and health (GMC, 2009a).

The GMC outcomes are similar to the CanMEDS 2005 (updated in 2015) framework of the Royal College of Physicians and Surgeons of Canada (Frank, 2005) (www.royalcollege.ca/portal/page/portal/rc/canmeds/framework), which has been adopted by other countries. It describes the core competencies required by doctors (medical experts) for better patient outcomes under seven roles: medical expert (central role), professional, scholar, communicator, collaborator, health advocate and manager.

# 10 Learning and teaching professionalism

- Knowledge of the various principles and methods you will encounter during professionalism education
- Definition and practice of reflection
- Learning through role play
- Learning through small group work
- Learning through experience

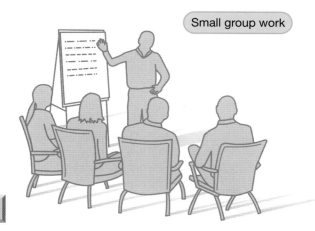

Small group work

University of Anycity Faculty of Health: professionalism module

| Date | Topic | Activity |
| --- | --- | --- |
| 12 October | The Hippocratic oath –relevance for today? | Lecture: The oath–history and format. Small group work–rewriting the oath for the 21st century |
| 19 October | Being a professional | Lecture–film & TV clips to stimulate discussion–small group work–good medical practice (or similar) |
| 26 October | Working with other professionals | Interprofessional learning sessions in small groups |
| 2 November | Reflection | What is reflection? Small group session and role play |
| 15 January | Observation in a clinical setting | Small group exercise and reflection |
| 22 January | Professionalism dilemmas | Small group discussion and reflection–input from patients and service users |
| 29 January | Working in health | Input from junior doctors/health professionals–discussion of learning from real life experiences–'what I wish I had known |

Role play

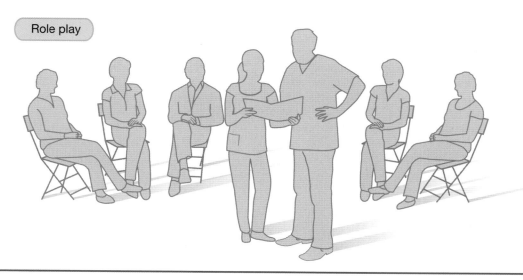

*Health Care Professionalism at a Glance*, First Edition. Jill Thistlethwaite and Judy McKimm.
© 2016 by John Wiley & Sons, Ltd. Published 2016 by John Wiley & Sons, Ltd.

We defined the formal curriculum in Chapter 9. In this chapter we look at various methods that medical schools have adopted to teach this formal curriculum and the educational principles they are based on. This should be helpful for you as many students consider these types of activities as somehow less useful or important than the science-based subjects you are learning in parallel with them.

Educators and clinicians have been debating the question of how to teach professionalism for many years. There are a lot of publications about professionalism, which your teachers read and consider as they develop and deliver the activities you undertake. Your formal curriculum probably has specific sessions devoted to ethics, medical law, teamwork and communication skills. There are likely to be other group work activities to promote discussion and reflection.

## Learning and teaching methods and principles

The timetabled learning activities should provide **context** and be **relevant** to clinical practice. So teaching should be grounded in the real world of patient interaction, your health service and the experiences that you and your peers are encountering or likely to encounter. This is why clinicians are often involved in the teaching — they bring their own examples of practice-based encounters and dilemmas — much more stimulating for all concerned.

Teaching and learning should also be based as much as possible on **your experiences.** To start with these may be your experiences as a patient, carer or observer of health professionals in action. Teachers may even use media portrayals of doctors and other health professionals as examples for discussion. When you begin to have patient contact and are immersed in clinical environments, you will have plenty of stories and experiences you want to discuss in professionalism sessions.

---

• Think of examples of a health professional's behaviour that you have observed that you would define as 'professional' and 'unprofessional'. How would you tell these stories to your peers? What may you and your peers learn from them?
• Now consider the portrayal of doctors in the media. Famous examples in TV programs are *House*, *Gray's Anatomy* and *Casualty*. There are also reality TV programmes that follow the working days of junior doctors and health care delivery in various real hospital settings. What can you learn about professionalism from such programmes?

---

## The importance of reflection

Thinking of examples as you did in the exercise above is not enough. Examples, your own and from observation, are *poor* teachers if you do not have the opportunity and guidance to reflect, particularly in relation to value conflicts and development of your self-awareness.

Reflection as a group exercise is thoughtful discussion. You can consider how you might behave in certain circumstances and the consequences of those actions. What would be the outcome if you did something differently? Self-reflection is also important but you will probably find reflection more helpful to start with as a group process as long as you and your colleagues are supportive and constructive in their criticism (see Chapter 19 for more on reflection).

## Example of a story to promote reflection

---

Maria, a first-year medical student, tells her group about going to see her GP when she was 15 because of irregular menstrual periods. Because of her age the receptionist insisted that Maria's mother go into the consulting room with her. During the consultation the GP hardly looked at Maria, he directed his questions to her mother and spent most of the time looking at his computer screen. When Maria did volunteer that her last period had been six weeks ago, the doctor said 'do you think you're pregnant?' Maria explained that she hadn't felt like visiting a GP again and hoped that she would be a better doctor.

---

In a small group session focussing on Maria's story, the facilitator will first thank Maria for volunteering to tell of her encounter. The facilitator may then ask Maria what would be most helpful for her to discuss in terms of the GP's professionalism. This might include
• Can (legal question)/should a doctor consult with a patient under the age of 16 years without a parent/guardian present?
• What communication skills did the doctor display and/or lack?
• How might a computer affect an interaction?
• Should the doctor have asked about the possibility of pregnancy?
• What would be a better way of doing this?
• What attributes of professionalism does this doctor need to improve?
• How might Maria become a 'better' doctor? What does this mean?

The facilitator may also suggest that three of the group role-play the consultation as Maria, her mother and the GP. Role-play is a common method of experiential learning. As a student you may at first be uncomfortable role-playing but if you overcome your embarrassment you will be able to look at events from different perspectives. You can experience how it feels to be unprofessional.

---

**Role-play** refers to two or more people taking on a different personality or carrying out actions in a scenario.

---

## The content of formal learning

It is impossible to have formal sessions for everything you need to know and be able to do as a health professional. Curriculum planners for professionalism outcomes look at the important issues that students and juniors will face frequently and build sessions round these, as well as use your experiences as outlined above. Common professionalism dilemmas include what to do after, for example, observing poor patient care, being abused as a student and lack of consent (see Rees et al., 2013, for teaching and learning relating to professionalism dilemmas: see Chapter 38 case scenarios).

# 11 Informal learning, role models and the hidden curriculum

**Menna Brown**

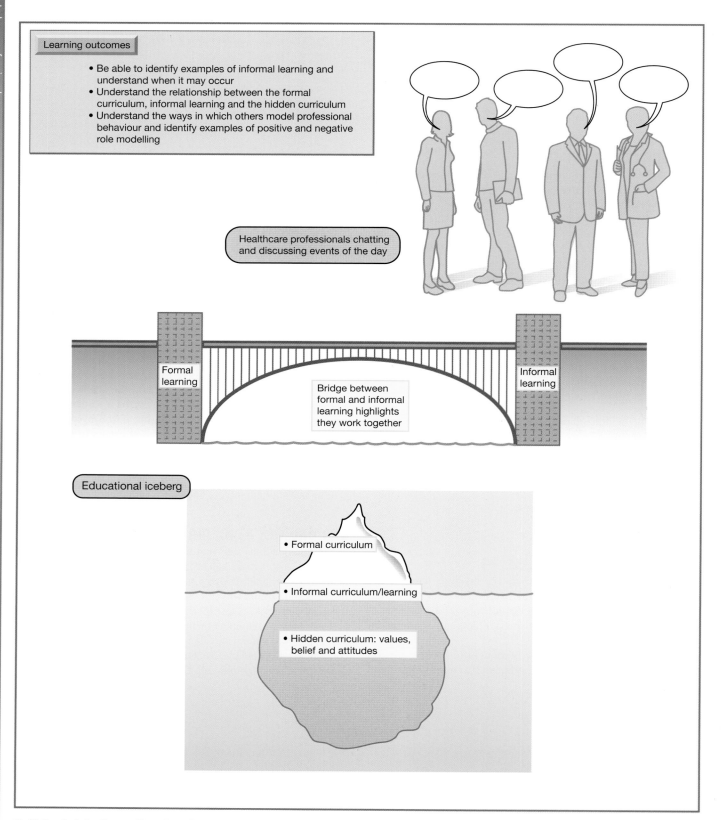

**Learning outcomes**

- Be able to identify examples of informal learning and understand when it may occur
- Understand the relationship between the formal curriculum, informal learning and the hidden curriculum
- Understand the ways in which others model professional behaviour and identify examples of positive and negative role modelling

Healthcare professionals chatting and discussing events of the day

Formal learning

Informal learning

Bridge between formal and informal learning highlights they work together

**Educational iceberg**

- Formal curriculum
- Informal curriculum/learning
- Hidden curriculum: values, belief and attitudes

*Health Care Professionalism at a Glance*, First Edition. Jill Thistlethwaite and Judy McKimm.

## Definition

'Informal learning is any activity involving the pursuit of understanding, knowledge or skill which occurs outside the curricula of educational institutions, or the courses or workshops offered by educational or social agencies.' Livingstone (1999, p. 51)

## Informal learning

Informal learning is a common term used in adult and postgraduate learning which refers to learning that occurs predominately in the workplace, the terms of which are determined by the individual, undertaken alone, without externally imposed criteria. This learning is flexible, free from the strict structures associated with formal learning and occurs without a teacher present. Learning can be thought of along a spectrum which ranges from 'unplanned and unintended' (informal) to 'deliberate and planned' (formal). It includes 'reactive' learning which is explicit but spontaneous.

Informal, work-based learning occurs in situations and settings outside formal education or teacher-led sessions. It occurs during interactions with others, from personal experiences and is often unintended. It is considered complementary to the formal curriculum and is largely invisible. As such it can often be taken for granted or assumed to have taken place and individuals may not always recognise when it has occurred (implicit learning). However, this is not always the case, for example an individual can undertake explicit informal learning through reflection and feedback, the retrospective recognition that learning has occurred and the identification that a new knowledge or skill has been learned through one's own processes (not through instruction by a teacher/instructor) (Eraut 2004).

Recent changes within continuing medical education have led to an increased emphasis on understanding the processes involved in informal learning including the way in which trainees become expert. Regulatory bodies involved in monitoring and supporting continuing medical education in the UK include the Medical Royal Colleges and Departments of Postgraduate Medical Education.

## Role models

A role model is a person whose behaviour, for example, or success is or can be emulated by others. Role models have been shown as a way to 'inculcate professional values, attitudes, and behaviours in students and young doctors' (Paice et al., 2002, p. 707).

The use of teaching staff as role models for professional behaviour has long been an informal part of medical training. The medical education literature documents the importance of role models in developing professional values, attitudes and character formation.

Important qualities in a role model include a positive attitude to junior colleagues, compassion for patients and integrity. Students choose traits from a variety of role models as opposed to one specific individual, positive and negative. However, many are often drawn to and emulate those with responsibility and status. Consultants involved with the educational supervision of doctors in training have a responsibility for role modelling the principles of good medical practice.

Three types of role modelling are described in the literature: (1) active identification; classic modelling and emulation of role models' behaviour, (2) active rejection and (3) inactive orientation; reinforcement of existing values. Identification with role models is considered by organisational behaviour theorists as critical to individual growth and development.

> Rosie, a medical student, observed Dr. Powell disregarding the opinion of Sian, a pharmacist, during a multi-disciplinary team meeting. How might this influence Rosie's actions in the future? What might she have learned from this encounter?

## Hidden curriculum

Hafferty and Franks (1994) described a multidimensional learning environment which takes into account three interrelated aspects of learning: (1) the stated, intended and formally endorsed curriculum (the formal curriculum); (2) interpersonal teaching and learning which occurs unplanned between staff and students (the informal curriculum) and (3) the transmission of norms, beliefs and values at the organisational, structural and cultural level (the hidden curriculum).

The hidden curriculum can be seen both as an underpinning or as a side-effect of the learning process. It is often considered with negative connotations although there are a number of associated positive influences: reinforcement of the formal curriculum, reinforcement of programme objectives and support for best practice activities. The hidden curriculum contrasts with the formal curriculum and is learned not through the processes of formal education but through implicit messages and social transmission. Commonly held understandings, values, beliefs and norms are conveyed through: staff and student relationships; disciplinary management or assessment systems; and policies and decisions communicated to the organisation and wider community. The effect of the hidden curriculum is to socialise the individual into the accepted organisational and cultural norms of society, a profession or an organisation. Students experience a sheltered version, compared to those in clinical practice who are exposed to the full societal context related to professional socialisation.

> Consider the different clinical environments where you have worked — for example, wards, hospital clinics and the community. How did they differ? What practices were promoted or discouraged? What did you learn from each?

# 12 Assessing professionalism

- Different methods of assessing professionalism
- The OSCE
- Workbased assessment
- The importance of feedback

**Example of item on MSF**
*Empathy and respect:*
Is polite, considerate and respectful to patients and colleagues of all levels; compassion and empathy towards patients and their relatives

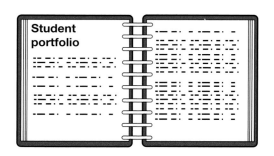

Student portfolio

**A portfolio** is a collection of a student's work that demonstrates the student's efforts, progress and achievements. It includes evidence of meeting learning outcomes and developing competencies.

You, the learner, should have a choice in what is included. There is usually an expectation of reflection on learning: how do you know you are competent? How have you demonstrated professional behaviour?

It will include forms such as mini-CEXs, MSFs and supervisors' reports. **A portfolio is** particularly useful for documenting personal and professional development.

It may form part of end-point (summative) assessment.

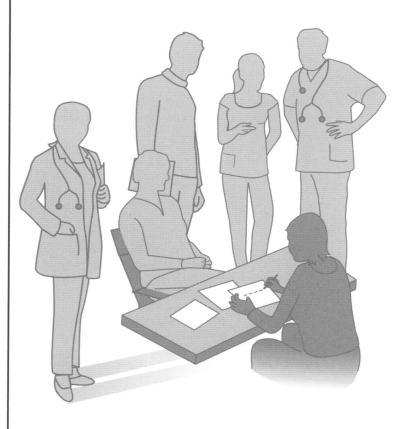

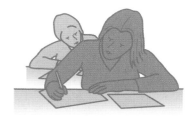

**Examples of items from a P-MEX**
- Solicited feedback
- Accepted feedback
- Addressed gaps in knowledge & skills
- Maintained patient confidentiality

**Examples of an SJT–for a medical student**
You are on a surgical rotation and have not yet carried out a breast examination except on a manikin and volunteer patient. On the ward the sugical registrar stops at a bed and asks each student to examine the patient's breasts. You are 8th in line. The patient is obviously becoming distressed. What do you do?
(You are given 4–5 options and have to rank them in order of appropriateness).

*Health Care Professionalism at a Glance*, First Edition. Jill Thistlethwaite and Judy McKimm.
© 2016 by John Wiley & Sons, Ltd. Published 2016 by John Wiley & Sons, Ltd.

# General principles

Just as aspects of professionalism and professional behaviour may be taught and learned, so too can aspects and behaviours be observed and assessed. As we have seen, professionalism is a multi-dimensional construct, dependent on cultural contexts, individuals, teams and situations. Therefore, unlike other parts of your curriculum, we cannot say to an individual: 'yes you have passed and are now competent as a professional'. The assessment of professional behaviour and attitudes needs to be longitudinal, and developmental, so observation and feedback are important. Of course, one or more incidences of unprofessional behaviour may lead to harsher sanctions than the need to sit an assessment again.

> Think of the various aspects of professionalism we have covered in this book and you have undertaken in your programme. What do you think are fair, feasible and equitable methods of assessment?

## What is being assessed?

The complexity of defining the attributes, competencies and behaviours that comprise 'professionalism' in practice means that assessments need to cover knowledge and understanding; practical skills/procedures; problem solving and behaviours that reflect attitudes. Behaviours must be assessed in context as you may act unprofessionally when you are under pressure to do so: for example, trying several times to perform a procedure because you need to practise. It is easier to behave well when you know you are being observed.

## Written assessment

Paper or computer-based tests can be used to test the knowledge or understanding which underpins professional practice.

*Case studies* involving patients/families/carers: these can be designed to explore how you link ethical principles and dilemmas to clinical practice or what a patient-centred approach would look like in certain circumstances. Some universities include family studies in the early years of a programme in which a student is attached to a family or patient over time to gain an understanding of how illness or disability changes, and how people live with these experiences. The assessment may be a journal or case history based on this longitudinal interaction with reflection on learning (see Chapter 19).

*Service improvement projects and audits* are frequently required and either hospital or community-based. They help you consider how and why health services change, put evidence-based practice into action and promote the role of the learner as a change champion.

*Multiple choice questions* (MCQs) *and essays* may also be used, although MCQs are difficult to write in this area. Essays are less commonly used, particularly for large numbers of students, as marking is labour-intensive. *Short answer questions* are sometimes included in written papers such as modified essay questions in which a case unfolds which involves a professionalism issue as well as the application of science and clinical knowledge.

*Situational judgement tests* (SJTs) are used more in selection for medical schools or postgraduate training (see Chapter 13). Learners have to rank their responses to professional dilemma-based scenarios. There is not usually one clear answer, but some are better (and worse) than others (see *The Situational Judgment Test at a Glance* in the same series as this).

## Group- or team-based assessment

As one way of learning professionalism is in facilitated discussion with peers, group-based learning and assessment is common. Your facilitator will be observing the interactions of the group, how members behave and what is said. There may be a mark for performance within the group over a year. You should be aware of how these marks are awarded and ideally your performance should be discussed with you to enhance learning. If anyone is performing badly, there should be a system of notification so that the learner can take steps to improve.

The patient or family cases or audits, etc. may be assessed through a group presentation, with marks for content and the process of the presentation itself. You may be asked to mark your peers and yourself to get an overall grade.

# Practical assessment

## The OSCE (objective structured clinical examination)

Practical skills-based assessments, whether of single competencies (e.g. examining the breasts) or multiple, complex high-level competencies (e.g. managing a cardiac arrest; dealing with an aggressive patient), are held under test conditions. Professional behaviour is one of the items under consideration. The most common assessment is the OSCE, in which stations test different competencies of varying levels of complexity. The examination is designed to test practical skills, written ability and verbal and non-verbal behaviours. Stations may include video or computer-based ethical scenarios as well as clinical and communication skills assessments with simulators, manikins, actors, simulated patients or real patients.

Examples of professionalism criteria:

- Introducing oneself
- Washing hands before and after patient contact
- Checking that the patient is comfortable
- Taking informed consent
- Being respectful
- Demonstrating empathy etc.

## Work-based assessment (WBA)

These are generally considered to be the most appropriate tests of professional practice when carried out on multiple occasions, by different observers, in different contexts and locations. Most programmes include an 'end of rotation' assessment of learners' performance completed by the supervising clinician and/or members of their team. This is usually a checklist which asks various questions relating to clinical abilities as well as how the learner worked with the team, with patients and families, their timekeeping, professionalism, etc. The P-MEX (professional mini-evaluation exercise) considers four sets of professional skills. The Mini-CEX focuses on specific aspects of clinical performance or observed clinical encounters and incorporates professional domains.

# Feedback and assessment

Ideally, all assessments should aim to encourage and facilitate learning and reflection through timely and constructive feedback. Optimal feedback focusses on improving performance or highlighting unhelpful behaviours, uses specific examples and is a dialogue between the learner and the observer. **Multisource (or 360-degree) feedback** (MSF) is a specific approach that gathers and collates standardised feedback from peers, colleagues, a range of professionals or patients in a systematic way. MSF is a powerful tool for development if used well but feedback should be given carefully and with support, especially if negative. Patient satisfaction surveys are becoming increasingly common for practising clinicians and, with MSF, are required for revalidation in the United Kingdom (Chapter 7).

**Principles of selection**

- The selection process
- Selecting for professional attributes
- The interview
- Multiple mini-interviews (MMIs)
- Situational Judgement Tests (SJTs)

### ANYTOWN MULTIPLE MINI INTERVIEW

**You have 8 minutes at each station, one minute to read the scenario and then the rest of the time to speak with the interviewer.**

**STATION 1**

*You are just about to go into a lecture where attendance is monitored when one of your friends asks you to sign in for them as they have to go to return an overdue library book.*
  *What do you say?*

**STATION 7**

*What attracted you to medicine?*
  *What are you most looking forward to in being a medical student and a doctor?*
  *If you don't get into medicine, what are your plans?*

**STATION 6**

*You are on placement with Dr Jan, a GP who tells you that he often gives antibiotics or other unnecessary medication to some patients 'because it makes them feel better and they expect me to give them medicine'.*
  *What do you think about Dr Jan's practice? What would you do, if anything?*

**STATION 2**

*You are on placement with a final year student who you'd heard on the grapevine has anorexia. You hear her vomiting in the toilets and when you ask her if she is OK, she says she is fine.*
  *Who do you speak to?*

**STATION 5**

*Tell us about a time when you found yourself in a dilemma.*
  *What was the dilemma, what issues did this raise for you and what did you do?*
  *What learning lessons did the experience give you?*

**STATION 3**

*Your second year case study project was with Annie, a terminally ill cancer patient. In the course of the project, you got very close to her and a few months later, you are informed that she has left you some money in her will 'in recognition of your care and compassion'.*
  *What issues does this identify? Is there a difference between being a student or a qualified doctor?*

**STATION 4**

*At this station you are asked to have a conversation with this patient (actor) for four minutes and find out six things about them. A bell will ring and then you will be asked to recall these and answer questions about them.*

*Health Care Professionalism at a Glance*, First Edition. Jill Thistlethwaite and Judy McKimm.
© 2016 by John Wiley & Sons, Ltd. Published 2016 by John Wiley & Sons, Ltd.

This chapter will describe some of the key features of the selection processes used for medical and health care professions.

# The selection process

Some sort of selection process is commonly used to recruit individuals into each of the various stages of education and training and for subsequent jobs as a fully qualified professional. Whilst selection processes differ depending on the stage of training or career, some common features exist and an understanding of the purpose and format of these can help you perform better. Because places/posts are limited and competition is usually fairly fierce, universities, postgraduate training organisations and healthcare organisations need to put a series of hurdles in place with the aim of finding the best person for the job. Although selectors are looking to predict potential or future performance, this is difficult to do and so a range of instruments are used. Selection processes typically consider a series of essential and desirable criteria based around:

• Academic or professional qualifications–do you meet the agreed level needed for the place/post?
• Skills or competencies–include practical skills (e.g. surgical competence) as well as 'softer' skills such as written and verbal communication or leadership
• Motivation, interest, enthusiasm for the place/post
• Aptitude for the role
• Views of other people who know you, for example, referees, teachers and deans

In order to assess the criteria, selection processes may involve written components, for example, application forms (including the 'open space' completed by applicants), an essay; evidence of past performance or tests; practical components such as an Objective Structured Clinical Examination (OSCE) or simulation; and evaluation of communication skills, for example, interview, engagement in social events, group activities and presentation. For some senior posts, these activities may take place over a number of days so that the organisation can get feedback from, and the opinion of, a wide range of potential colleagues.

> Think about the last time you applied for a place/post. How well do you think the activities you engaged in assessed the knowledge, skills and qualities needed for the position?

# Interviews

Interviews are usually carried out face-to-face (or via video conference or telephone) with the applicant answering a series of structured questions from two or more people aimed at identifying their strengths, motivation, understanding of the organisation/post and how well they communicate. Sometimes applicants will be required to give a presentation, for example, on what they see as the challenges of the role. Although interviews have been criticised for being selective, subject to interviewer bias, unreliable and lacking in validity, they do give opportunity to meet candidates and see them in action.

# Selecting for professional attributes

It is relatively straightforward for organisations to be certain that applicants have the required academic and professional qualifications and that they are trained to a certain level (e.g. through graduation certificates or postgraduate college membership examinations). Aptitude tests, such as the UKCAT (UK Clinical Aptitude Test) and tests for verbal or numerical ability and reasoning have been shown to have predictive ability for future success in medical school (McManus et al., 2013).

The application form, interview, references and written tests can help provide some information, certainly enough to screen out those who do not meet threshold standards. However, in medicine and health care, it is vital that the organisations appointing individuals can be as assured as possible that they have the desired professional attributes, but this is much harder to ascertain and predict. Of course, if someone has been subject to criminal proceedings or disciplinary or fitness to practise procedures, then a red flag will be raised. But for the vast majority of applicants (particularly those applying to medical school) it is very challenging to select for professional attributes such as integrity, honesty, compassion, teamworking or coping under pressure. In order to address this, new selection methods have been introduced including psychometric tests and group activities. Two of the most widely used additional selection methods are described below.

# Situational judgement tests

The situational judgement test (SJT) is now used for selection to the UK Foundation programme (i.e. the first two years after graduation) and for some medical schools (as well as in selection for many other professions such as teaching). It is a written multiple choice test in which candidates have to select which they think is the best response to a dilemma-based scenario. The aim of the SJT is to identify applicants who might lack elements of professional judgement.

# Multiple mini interviews

Multiple mini interviews (MMIs) have been used in selection to medicine for a number of years. Based on the design of the OSCE, MMIs require candidates to move around a series of 10–12 brief 'stations' (e.g. 5–10 minutes) at which one or two interviewers ask questions based on previous experiences, defined situations or practical tests. Eva and Macala (2014) describe this situation in one station:

> You are in your first year of medicine. In your PBL (problem-based learning) group of five students, you are encouraged to share your knowledge, teach each other, and contribute to the discussion. However, you notice that one of your colleagues is often quiet, shy and participates very little in the discussion. He also appears to do the minimum required work and his lack of participation is causing problems for the group. What would you do in this situation? (p. 607)

Although test content differs depending on the organisation and its goals, both the SJT and MMI provide a means of assessing a range of professional attributes including coping with pressure, effective communication, learning and professional development, organisation and planning, patient focus, problem solving and decision-making, self-awareness and insight and working effectively as part of a team.

# 14 Academic writing and plagiarism

## George Ridgway

**Figure. 14.1** Levels of plagiarism

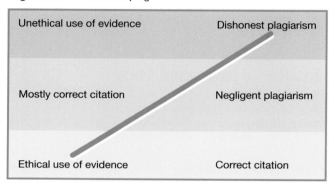

**Figure. 14. 2** The importance of evidence in supporting propositions

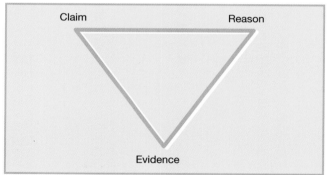

**Figure. 14. 3** Methods of information transfer

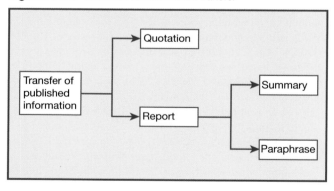

**Figure. 14. 4** Reporting verbs and the writer's opinion of evidence

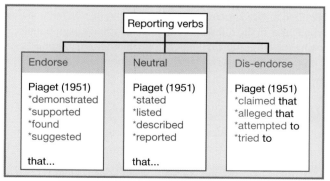

*Health Care Professionalism at a Glance*, First Edition. Jill Thistlethwaite and Judy McKimm.
© 2016 by John Wiley & Sons, Ltd. Published 2016 by John Wiley & Sons, Ltd.

# What is plagiarism?

Transferring ideas, findings or works as evidence in your own writing (papers, assignments, etc.) incorrectly or without properly acknowledging the original source is plagiarism. There are different levels of plagiarism, which can be shown as an incline of degree of seriousness (Fig. 14.1), ranging from accidental to deliberate plagiarism. While accidental plagiarism might be due to negligence or poor referencing practices it can seriously undermine the validity of possible claims made in a paper. Plagiarism is unprofessional at any level from student to clinician to academic.

## The research triangle

When writing a research paper for a journal or assignment, the strength of your arguments will be based on the research triangle. First you will be making one or more **claims**. A claim is a proposition that can be argued as true or false, or even perhaps as partly true or partly false. Consider the claim: 'The doctor who prefers compliant patients is usually practising in a paternalistic manner'. To convince the reader you need to provide a **reason** to support the claim. One reason could be 'because paternalism relies on a relationship based on unequal power'. To convince your readers, the reason needs the support of **evidence** derived from a reliable source such as the *British Medical Journal*. The success of convincing the reader about the claim depends on linking each of the three parts. The importance of evidence in supporting a claim and reason pairing propositions is shown in Figure 14.2.

You can provide evidence, but it will not be valid unless it has itself been published in a reliable format such as a peer-reviewed journal, conference proceedings, report from a respected organisation in the field or academic book. Once evidence has been published it can be used to support the claims in your paper by transfer from these sources through quoting, summarising or paraphrasing the author(s) of the evidence as shown in Figure 14.3.

## Dishonest plagiarism

According to the University of Sydney Academic Dishonesty and Plagiarism in Coursework Policy (2012), dishonest plagiarism means knowingly using 'another person's work as one's own work by presenting, copying or reproducing it without appropriate acknowledgement of the source' (p. 5). While negligent plagiarism resulting from the careless transfer of information may require the paper to be resubmitted, a paper containing dishonest plagiarism may be rejected. Dishonest plagiarism in assignments will result in a fail and potentially in expulsion from your degree. (Check your own university's policy and guidelines.) Consequently writers must have confidence in knowing when and how to transfer information into their paper by quoting, summarizing or paraphrasing.

# Referencing other people's work

**Quoting** a source means that you have a reason to focus on the author of the transferred information at least as much as the information. This may be to acknowledge an author who is considered an important expert authority on the topic, or who has phrased information with particular clarity. This type of citation is used to focus on the author and the author's text and requires you to follow strict rules for quotation. If the quotation has fewer than 40 words, integrate it into the text and enclose the quotation with double quotation marks. For quotations of more than 40 words start a new indented paragraph. A quote must be accompanied by the authors' names (and page number in certain reference conventions) and bibliographical details provided in a reference list usually at the end of the paper. The use of long quotations and diagrams/figures also requires permission for reproduction from the copyright holder – normally the publisher of the work you wish to use.

> **Example of a direct quote**
> 'According to a survey published by the Freshminds recruitment consultancy, as many as one in four university students may have cheated by copying material for essays from the internet'. (Eaton, 2004, p.70)
> Reference: Eaton L. (2004). A quarter of UK students are guilty of plagiarism survey shows. *BMJ*, 329, 70.

Quotation should be used sparingly, however, as overuse will result in a text with too much focus on the quoted author and too much repetition of the author's words. This leads to a form of negligent plagiarism in which the writer becomes dependent on the quoted author's understanding of information by failing to express the information in a novel manner.

**Paraphrasing** is the type of information transfer which allows the writer great freedom of expression and control over the focus of information. If the writer keeps to the same meaning of information expressed in the original text, then a new combination of words can be assembled to transfer the information. The writer can choose to focus on the author of the information or the information itself (termed author prominent and information citation, respectively). Author prominent citation requires a reporting verb, which can inform the reader whether the evidence is endorsed, dis-endorsed or considered as neutral by the writer. In other words the writer's opinion of the author's evidence can be made explicit. A range of reporting verbs is shown in Figure 14.4. Good writers can paraphrase a text by re-writing it in their own words so that it carries the same meaning. Not knowing how to paraphrase a text can lead to plagiarism because the writer does not re-phrase it.

> **Example of a paraphrase**
> The first example is a direct quote and the second is paraphrased.
> 1. 'Half the students (54%) summarised their sources incorrectly, either by directly copying the words of the source or by failing to communicate what the source had reported in the summary; 13% of the students did not provide reference details for the source and 32% gave incomplete details' (Joubert et al., 2009, p. 1090).
> 2. Joubert et al. (2009) found summaries of sources were inaccurately written by half the students (54%), due to the direct reproduction of the original material, or failure to communicate the original meaning, while 13% of the students provided no reference to the original material and 32% supplied inadequate references.
> *Try paraphrasing the Eaton quote above.*

**Summarising** an author follows the same general principles but much less of the information in the original text is transferred. It tends to be used where there is general agreement on the information.

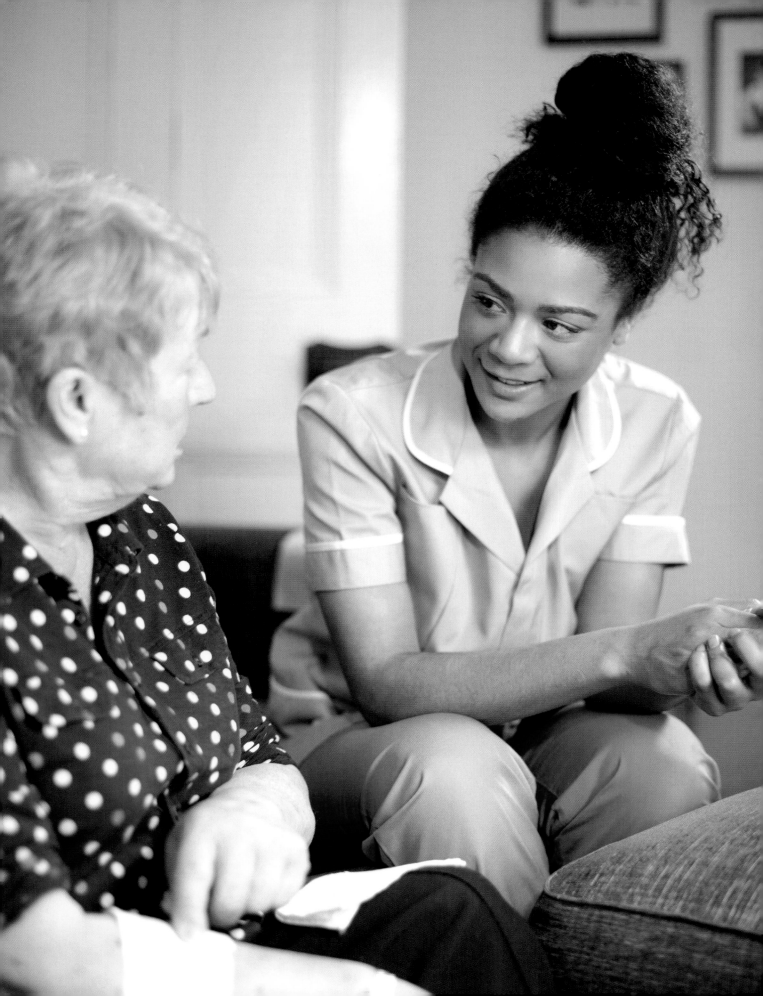

# Professionalism in practice

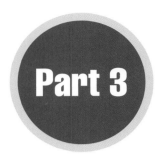

**Part 3**

## Chapters

# 15 Professional behaviours

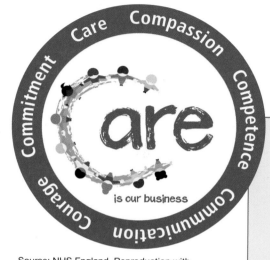

Source: NHS England. Reproduction with permission of NHS England.

## Professional behaviours for quality care
### 'A culture of compassionate care'

The UK's National Health Service (NHS) focuses on its staff delivering high quality care to all its patients and having 'the right staff, with the right skills, in the right place'.
NHS England defines the key elements of NHS culture as the '6Cs':

1 **Care**–is the core business for individuals and communities and people have a right for this to be provided throughout all stages of life
2 **Compassion**–care given through relationships based on empathy, respect and dignity–'kindness'
3 **Competence**–understanding people's health and social needs and having the expertise to deliver evidence based care
4 **Communication**–central to caring relationships and team working and for 'no decision about me without me'
5 **Courage**–to do the right thing, to speak out and to innovate and embrace new ways of working
6 **Commitment**–to patients and populations to improve care and experiences

Source:
www.england.nhs.uk/wp-content/uploads/2012/12/6c-a5-leaflet.pdf

All health professionals are expected to behave 'professionally', but what does this mean in practice and do we (or should we) expect the same standards of behaviour from students as practising professionals?

## Professional attributes and behaviours

Desirable professional attributes of health professionals are closely linked to personal and cultural values as displayed in practice. There is some consistency globally around such attributes which include leadership, good communication, trustful and respectful relationships, honesty, integrity, empathy, compassion, care and 'patient-centredness'. However, in the process of becoming professional, such attributes can be modified in positive (acquired) and negative (attrition) ways through experiences in both education and work environments (Hilton and Slotnick, 2005).

Hafferty (2004) reminds us that professional attributes need to be translated into operational and observable practices and behaviours. Such behaviours are the public, outward facing demonstration of professionalism and are the main ways in which professionalism is taught and assessed (see Chapters 10-12).

## Proto-professionalism

Hilton and Slotnik (2005) suggest that whilst aspiring or current students might display some of the elements of professionalism, it is only through the acquisition of 'phronesis' (practical wisdom) over time that an individual becomes a truly mature 'professional'. They describe the long timeframe over which such practical wisdom is developed as the period of 'proto-professionalism'. During this period, the proto-professionals need to develop the individual attributes of ethical practice, reflection and responsibility and the collaborative attributes of teamworking, social responsibility and respect for patients. Individuals are always learning and developing practical wisdom throughout their lives through reflection on different experiences and situations.

## Personality factors

Understanding one's (and others') personality types and preferences can help in the development of more effective communication skills and explain why people behave as they do. A number of instruments and models have been used in studies on health professionals including Transactional Analysis models, 'Big Five' or 'Five factor' tests and Jungian type scales. For example, Clack et al.'s (2004) study using the Myers Briggs Type Indicator® (MBTI®) found that there were differences between doctors and the wider UK population, particularly in the way information was taken in and how learning occurred. This has implications for possible

miscommunication. Learning more about yourself and gaining self-insight, as personalities are not necessarily static, can help you modify your behaviours and approaches to different patients, colleagues and situations.

## Mindful practice

Epstein (1999) suggests that one of the key elements of professionalism is that of 'mindful practice', which underpins critical self-reflection. The characteristics of mindful practice are

- 'Active observation of oneself, the patient and the problem
- Peripheral vision
- Pre-attentive processing
- Critical curiosity
- Courage to see the world as it is rather than as one would have it be
- Willingness to examine and set aside categories and prejudices
- Adoption of a beginner's mind
- Humility to tolerate awareness of one's areas of incompetence
- Connection between the knower and the known
- Compassion based on insight
- Presence'

Epstein describes five levels of mindfulness, ranging from level 0 (denial and externalisation) through developing curiosity and self-insight to level 5 (generalisation, incorporation and presence). Keeping reflective journals, receiving feedback and critical/significant event reports help develop clinical practice. Mindfulness goes further: it involves 'reflection in action' and clinicians modelling moment-to-moment awareness of their knowledge and decision-making processes, making overt and explicit what are often tacit, internal, subconscious processes. This is a discipline and attitude of mind rather than a learned set of behaviours, requiring support and mentoring, as it can be emotionally difficult.

## Belief systems and social responsibility

Wynia et al. (2014) note that using simple checklists of behaviours poses the risk that learners can be 'signed off' as being professional. They suggest professionalism is a belief system through which any profession can fulfil shared promises to the public about the delivery of health care. Professional behaviours and values are derived from this belief system rather than being the driving force. Professionals therefore need to engage in debate and dialogue as well as adhere to and co-create belief systems that underpin health care delivery.

The idea of social responsibility and social justice being part of professionalism is indicated in many frameworks and standards and is reflected in the increasing emphasis on the contribution of individuals and professional groups to developing and sustaining the right culture within organisations.

# 16 Empathy, compassion and altruism

Learning outcomes:

- Definitions of empathy, compassion and altruism
- The importance of empathy, compassion and altruism in clinical practice
- Reflection on how to recognise and develop these attributes

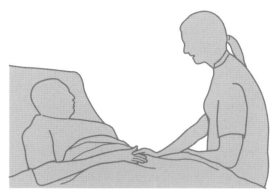

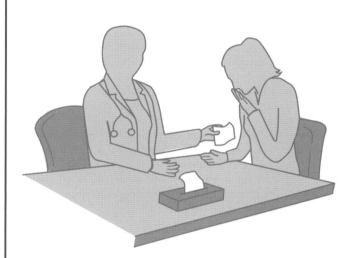

**Doctor as professional:**
1.1. Exhibit appropriate professional behaviours in practice, including honesty, integrity, commitment, compassion, respect and altruism

**Doctor as communicator:**
1.2. Establish positive therapeutic relationships with patients and their families that are characterised by understanding, trust, respect, honesty and empathy

**Doctor as expert:**
1.5. Demonstrates compassionate and patient-centered care

*Outcomes from the CanMEDS framework*

*Health Care Professionalism at a Glance*, First Edition. Jill Thistlethwaite and Judy McKimm.
© 2016 by John Wiley & Sons, Ltd. Published 2016 by John Wiley & Sons, Ltd.

# Definitions

*Empathy* is defined in a number of ways. The Oxford Dictionary states that it is 'the ability to understand and share the feelings of another'. To this we can also add identification with another's motives. An expert on 'empathic intelligence' defines empathy as 'the ability to understand your own thoughts and feelings and, by analogy, apply your self-understanding to the service of others, mindful that their thinking and feeling might not match your own' (Arnold, 2005). Contrast these definitions with sympathy: feeling pity and sorrow for someone else's misfortune. So empathy is more than a sympathetic feeling–it involves understanding and showing one's understanding. It is a more active process.

*Compassion* is the desire to enhance the well-being of others.

*Altruism* is the unselfish concern for the well-being of others. Altruism is therefore about **acting** on the feeling of compassion, though in a clinical situation this may also be referred to as compassionate care. Altruism is about action without thought of reward, for example: giving to charity, volunteering to work without pay for those less fortunate, waiving a fee if the patient cannot pay.

We can link the three by saying that altruism is triggered by empathy and driven by compassion.

> Think how these three attributes relate to professionalism. How might you recognise each in practice? Have they been mentioned in your programme so far? If you have observed doctors and nurses you may have seen acts of compassion. You may have seen a lack of compassion; such behaviour could be defined as unprofessional.

## Empathy

Can you ever really understand the feelings of another?

> Gita Patel is a junior nurse working in a hospital in a deprived area of a large town. She is speaking to a 35-year-old woman in the Emergency Department who has been admitted following an overdose of anti-depressant tablets. The patient, Clare, says she has not been able to get over the death of her younger brother and today is the second anniversary of the car accident in which he was killed. Gita says 'I can understand how difficult this must be for you'. Clare replies 'How can you understand? You don't have to live with missing him every day'. In fact, Gita's brother died at the age of 4 years from meningitis. She does not know how to respond, as she does not think it appropriate to mention her own feelings. On reflection, she does realise that every person's story is unique. When she talks over the incident with her supervisor he suggests a better empathic reply would be: 'I can see that this is very distressing for you'. This acknowledges that you are listening to the patient without claiming you know exactly how she feels.

You will learn about empathic responses in communication skill courses. They are more than words; they are also demonstrating understanding and checking its accuracy.

There are frequent reports that medical students lose empathy during their training; and female students have been shown to have higher empathy scores than men (see for example Chen et al., 2012). Reasons for this may include stress, tiredness, concentration on learning knowledge rather than interpersonal skills, lack of suitable role models and desensitisation to suffering as a survival tactic. It is important to take stock of your feelings regularly: are you showing signs of not caring anymore? Are the patients just a collection of clinical signs? Your professional development time should be a chance to talk about this and to reconnect with your humanity; discussion with your peers and sharing difficult interactions and situations will help. If you have a clinical mentor, this is someone else to talk to about your concerns.

Is empathy always a positive attribute? Is it possible to be too empathic so that a doctor loses professional detachment and is unable to act objectively? Do you think that good clinical practice and decision-making depends on a doctor being remote and unemotional? Is there a difference in how a doctor and nurse should behave in certain situations? It is all about degree and where on the continuum between totally detached and emotionally encumbered you want and need to be at a particular time. During a cardiac arrest you want to be 'professional' and think about the task in hand rather than the suffering of the patient and family. If the patient dies, the family would expect compassion and acknowledgement of their grief (see Chapter 17 for more on dealing with emotions).

## Compassion

'Medical care without compassion cannot be truly patient-centred' (Lown et al., 2011, p. 1172). Even though compassion is a feeling, there are acts which do demonstrate compassion to others: touching a patient's hand when you see he or she is in distress, lowering your voice when asking about painful episodes, responding when asked to do something distasteful with a smile rather than a grimace. Though difficult, sitting in silence at a patient's bedside because you have recognised their suffering shows care rather than rushing off when your shift is over. Compassion is about making connections between the patient and the professional.

## Compassion and altruism

Compassion fatigue is common in doctors in training who work long hours, who need to study and who have trouble adapting to the responsibility of their clinical role. While the public may expect that nurses are more caring than doctors, all health professionals should be able to connect with patients. The founder of the Schwartz foundation for compassionate health care said: 'the smallest acts of kindness make the unbearable bearable' (https://www.theschwartzcenter.org).

Compassion and altruism are more likely to be sustained if health professionals feel supported and recognised in their workplaces by managers and their colleagues (Jones, 2002). A simple thank you from a senior professional or a compliment from a patient for a job well done works wonders for self-esteem.

# 17 Handling emotions

Learning outcomes:

- Showing appropriate emotions
- Emotional labour
- Emotional intelligence (EI)
- Resilience, stress and burnout
- Seeking support

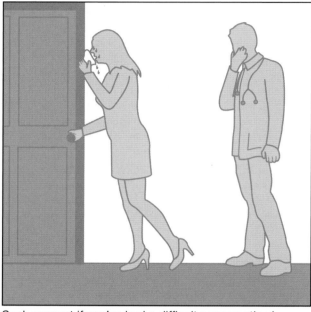

Seek support if you've had a difficult conversation/experience

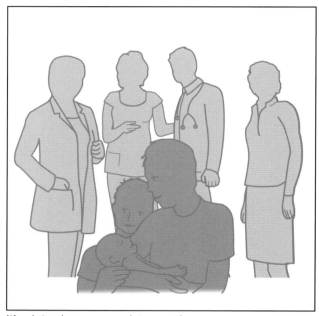

It's ok to show appropriate emotions

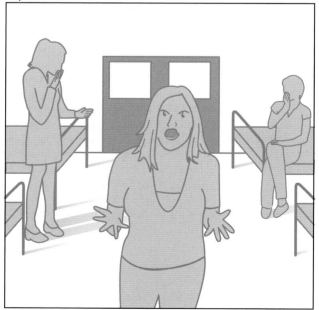

Learn how you behave when you're stressed

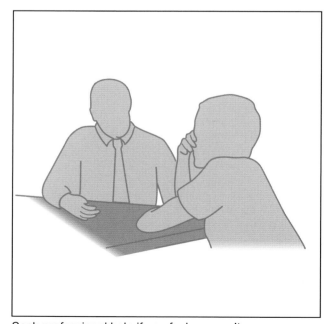

Seek professional help if you feel you can't cope

*Health Care Professionalism at a Glance*, First Edition. Jill Thistlethwaite and Judy McKimm.
© 2016 by John Wiley & Sons, Ltd. Published 2016 by John Wiley & Sons, Ltd.

Health and social care professionals work directly with people, often in situations of high emotion. 'People work' has long been acknowledged as taking an emotional toll on health workers. Learners and practitioners have to learn how to manage their own and others' emotions and 'act the part' without appearing too hard and objective or so affected by others' distress that they cannot function in their professional role. Everyone is different in how they react and respond to different emotional situations, patients and families, which is frequently linked to our own life experiences or upbringing.

---

Rakesh, a first year medical student on his first clinical placement watched as the two nurses gently settled Mr. Barnes, a dying, elderly man onto his pillows, dimmed the lights and closed the door behind them all to leave him and his wife of 60 years alone. He felt tears welling in his eyes and felt embarrassed.

They went into the office. Sarah, the young staff nurse, gave him a quick hug. Rakesh thanked her and said '*It's strange, but he reminded me of my grandfather when he died ...*'. She said '*it's OK, we all feel this, particularly with certain patients, I use these feelings to provide the best care I can. Although we're here to do a job it doesn't mean we don't feel people's distress*'. Mark, the student nurse, added '*what I was told on my first ward was to treat every patient as you would want your family member to be treated*'. Rakesh nodded, it seemed that even though Mr. Barnes was dying in hospital, they were doing all they could to make it a 'good death'. Talking this over with his flatmates later, he realised he had just learned some important lessons:
- You can show emotion but it needs to be appropriate
- Talking about how you feel helps you to understand how to deal with emotions
- Colleagues can provide good support, you are not on your own
- Always treat patients as you would want your family to be treated

---

## Emotional labour

'Emotional labour' is when paid work requires someone to express and regulate their own and others' emotions as part of their everyday work. Learning rapport, mirroring, reflecting and other communication skills are all part of developing and maintaining connections with people (patients as well as colleagues) and can help you manage your own emotions. A safe working environment 'contains' strong or difficult emotions through appropriate responses or strategies. For example, in emergency or rapidly deteriorating situations, a patient's family members are best looked after away from the bedside so that their strong emotions do not distract the health care team. When patients or carers are joyful, in pain, dying, distressed, frightened or angry, as a professional you need to know how to respond personally and as part of a team.

## Emotional Intelligence

Emotional Intelligence (EI) has been defined as '*a type of social intelligence that involves the ability to monitor one's own and others' emotions, to discriminate among them and to use this information*

*to guide one's own thinking and actions*' (Mayer and Salovey, 1997). It helps explain why some individuals are more capable than others of processing emotional information and using it to guide their behaviour. Mayer et al. (2003) later refined the construct to encompass the abilities to

1 Perceive emotions–detecting and reading emotions in self, in faces, pictures, voices, etc.
2 Use emotions in thinking and problem solving
3 Understand emotions in language, perceive nuance and track emotions over time
4. Regulate emotions in self and others.

Understanding your own EI can help you develop greater awareness and skills in handing emotions, problem solving and teamwork.

## Resilience, stress and burnout

An important attribute for health professionals is psychological resilience. Resilience is the ability to cope with stress and adversity by utilising effective and appropriate coping strategies and personal strengths. Many studies (e.g. Shanafelt and Dyrbye, 2012) emphasise that high workload, a loss of empathy and a constant need to manage difficult emotions all contribute to doctors' and other health professionals' stress and burnout. Whilst we all need a certain amount of positive stress to motivate and challenge us, when our usual coping strategies do not work, this can lead to problems.

Positive coping strategies include a healthy lifestyle, exercise, socialising, meditating and getting away from work or study. 'Comfort tricks' (e.g. drinking alcohol, overeating, smoking, withdrawal) may help in the short term, but if they become unhelpful habits or addictions, they are potentially dangerous. Continual high stress can lead to long-term physical or mental health problems or burnout. It is important when thinking about longer term career plans to consider what sort of stress actually motivates you and what is hard to cope with–everyone is different (see Chapter 18 on self-care).

## What can help?

- Purposefully observe how other professionals respond and deal with emotional situations.
- Be 'reflectively aware' of your own emotional responses, acknowledge them and ask whether these are appropriate. How might you regulate them if needed?
- Engage in activities to gain self-insight, learn what your strengths are and develop coping strategies (e.g. through supervision, debriefings, peer support groups, Balint groups)
- Ask for feedback and advice from others on how you behave–what you are feeling inside may (or may not) be apparent
- Learn how you behave when you're stressed–what coping strategies are helpful and what are not
- Career counselling can help you match your personality to the right context or specialty
- Seek professional help if you are feeling overwhelmed and that you cannot cope through your GP or counselling services

# 18 Self-care: looking after your own health

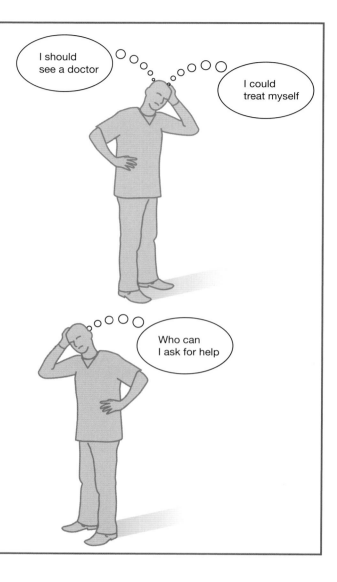

**Learning outcomes:**

- What to do when you are sick–as a student and later as a doctor
- The imposter syndrome
- Definition of burnout–prevention and treatment
- Where to seek help

Sunil Ghosh is a final year medical student who has an important assessment in two days time. He wakes up with a terrible sore throat, dry cough and runny nose. He feels he doesn't have the time to try to get a GP appointment and considers his options. Sunil suspects he has a viral infection but decides that antibiotics are worth a go to get him better for his exam. He could ring his dad, a paediatrician, and ask him to write a prescription, or he could ask his flatmate for the rest of her packet of antibiotics. She had an infection a while ago and didn't finish all her pills.
    What do you think Sunil should do and why?

- Feeling tired/tired all the time
- Not wanting or dreading going to work
- A sense of doom
- Poor communication with patients and peers
- Resenting or feeling hostile to patients
- Difficulty caring for others
- Working too quickly or too slowly
- Feeling tearful
- Anger towards team members
- Feeling put upon or the hardest worker in the team
- Taking time off work
- Feeling that what you do is useless
- Feelings related to the 'imposter syndrome'

**Symptoms of burnout**

*Health Care Professionalism at a Glance*, First Edition. Jill Thistlethwaite and Judy McKimm.
© 2016 by John Wiley & Sons, Ltd. Published 2016 by John Wiley & Sons, Ltd.

The famous physician Sir William Osler wrote:

*A doctor who treats him or herself has a fool for a doctor and an idiot for a patient.*

Yet doctors do continue to self-diagnose and treat themselves. They also neglect their own health and miss warning signs of illness. Being professional means seeking advice from the right professional at the right time. Corridor consultations, the quick word of advice given outside a formal consultation, are not appropriate. Ill doctors do not provide optimal care. Moreover they may spread disease by continuing to work when contagious. No one wants their health professional coughing into a wound. There is a tension between self-care and altruism. Doctors need to follow their own advice about sleep, physical exercise and healthy eating. But long hours and frequently stressful working conditions may hamper the desire to have an optimal life style.

## The sick doctor

Being a health professional is a stressful occupation. The British Medical Association (BMA) found that about one in fifteen doctors during their lifetimes become dependent on drugs or alcohol (BMA, 1998) with similar data published for Australian doctors (Khong et al., 2002). The proportion of doctors who suffer from higher levels of stress is about 28%, compared to 18% in the general working population (Firth-Cozens, 2003), and burnout is common.

Mental health is adversely affected because of the complex nature of the job with high stress impinging on personal lives and the frequent need to cope with uncertainty. Doctors often work long hours and have access to addictive drugs, which they use to help them relax after their busy days. Many doctors are married to doctors or other health professionals–the couples talk 'shop' and both partners may find it difficult to help each other unwind. Taking time off work can be regarded as a sign of weakness: 'I don't want to put extra pressure on my colleagues or let down my patients'. These thoughts turn into one of feeling indispensable and soon may lead to burnout.

## The sick student

We are sure you are aware that you and your peers as medical students are high achievers. You are often perfectionists. Most of your peers will never have failed an examination before coming to university and are used to being at the top of the class. But you cannot all be top. Failure is not something you will be familiar with and not doing well in examinations can be devastating for some.

The **imposter syndrome** is a collection of symptoms, which includes feeling inadequate even though you may continue to do well in your course. If affected you may have chronic self-doubt coupled with the worry that you are not qualified to be at medical school (or later to be a doctor) and that someone will find you out. Many medical students and doctors appear to have varying degrees of this condition. One study found that nearly one-third of respondents (medical, dental, nursing and pharmacy students) had experienced imposter syndrome (Henning et al., 1998). The symptoms are strongly correlated with diagnoses of anxiety and depression (Oriel et al., 2004).

**Burnout:** Physical and/or emotional exhaustion due to prolonged stress or frustration (see fig. 18.1). How would you rate your physical and mental health? What support does your medical school provide to help? What should it provide? Personal and professional development courses often cover self-care and what to do when you are ill. Have you registered with a GP or family doctor?

## Seeking help

The clear message from the GMC (2013b) and other accreditation bodies is that doctors should not diagnose or treat themselves or their families. Below are important considerations for doctors: they are old but still in force.

---

- It is not advisable for doctors to assume responsibility for the diagnosis and management of their own health problems or those of their immediate family, except in the most unusual circumstances.
- All doctors should be registered with a GP.
- As with all other patients, the responsibility for overall care and continuity of treatment for doctors and their families should rest with their GP. Referral for consultant advice or care should be made through their GP.
- It is not advisable for doctors to prescribe themselves anything other than over-the-counter (OTC) medicines.
- Doctors need to be aware that they become the patient in the doctor–patient relationship when they are receiving medical care.
- Doctors have an ethical duty to themselves and to their patients to ensure that their own health problems are effectively managed: to seek competent professional advice particularly on their ability to work and to follow this advice.

Adapted from British Medical Association, 1995.

---

Poor professional help-seeking behaviour starts early in medical school. A US study of 1027 students from nine medical schools found that 90% felt they had needed health care during medical school. However, over one-third found it difficult to access health care because of being too busy to take time off, and 15% had worries about confidentiality. Worryingly, two-thirds of the students had obtained informal care from colleagues and half had asked a colleague to perform a physical examination (Roberts et al., 2000). Medical students report barriers to seeking help about their health, being likely to seek advice informally from friends and/or family in regard to mental health care (Brimstone et al., 2007).

## Education and prevention

In your professionalism courses you may be discussing alcohol misuse and issues relating to prescribed and illegal drugs. Many medical students establish heavy drinking patterns early on in their careers. Universities have cheap alcohol and social life often revolves around student bars. Students who do not drink alcohol are often marginalized by this culture causing poor teamworking.

Your university should advise you where to seek confidential help and who provides support if you are stressed or depressed. It is common for students when learning about symptoms and diseases to think they have some awful condition. Many ignore these worries–but some conditions are genuine. Seek professional advice if you are unsure. Talking with others in de-briefing sessions or informally with colleagues will help relieve stress and make you aware of how working with patients affects professionals.

# 19 Reflective practice

- Definitions
- Purpose of reflection
- Written reflection
- The professional conversation
- Feedback

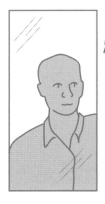
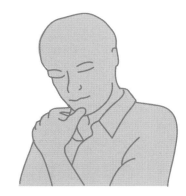
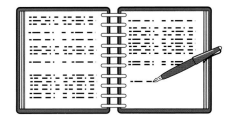

| More than simply looking in the mirror... | Deep thinking is required... | Written reflection can be helpful ... |
|---|---|---|
| I can see that Mr Morgan is very upset about his wife's deterioration. I think I'll leave the family for a little while to come to terms with what is happening and come back later | I know I rushed through that history taking and Dr Price's feedback reinforced that. Tonight I am going to practise the sequence so I am more rehearsed and ask Dr Price to observe me again tomorrow and ask her to slow me down if I go too fast or miss anything out | I was pleased with the way I managed to explain to Saha's parents about how her diagnosis of diabetes will affect her. I think I explained clearly and simply without being too patronising and they know to come back to me if they want to know more |
| Reflection on action | Reflection on action | Reflection on action |

## Definitions

A number of definitions of 'reflection' exist. These range from what Moon (2004) calls 'common sense reflection'–this is the day-to-day thinking we do after a situation has affected us–to 'critical reflection', which is a purposeful, questioning approach which requires us to challenge preconceived notions or ways of working (our 'taken for granted assumptions', Crawley, 2005). Other writers, including Schön (1983), have described four types of reflection that define professionals' behaviours:

• Reflection before action–this is reflective planning before you engage in an activity or situation;
• Reflection in action–this is reflecting on what is happening and your reactions 'in the moment', enabling you to change your practice or responses in an intuitive manner;
• Reflection on action–this is retrospective thinking about events that have already happened;
• Reflection for action–this is purposeful reflection aimed at defining new goals or learning.

## The purpose of reflection

The main purpose of reflection is to improve our practice and learn from experiences. We do this both for ourselves–to learn more about ourselves and how we work–but increasingly learners are also required to engage in reflection as a formal part of the curriculum or training programme. This can cause tensions, particularly if you feel you are just 'going through the motions'. It is therefore useful to think about the purpose of any reflection as this can help you decide how to approach it and what you (and others) might get out of it.

## How do we do it?

Boud et al. (1989) suggest three components that are involved in reflection: returning to an experience (recalling significant events), attending to or connecting with the feelings associated with the experience, and evaluating the experience in the light of existing knowledge or new understanding. It is important to think about feelings with a view to recognising helpful and unhelpful reactions as this will help you in future.

---

When he came on duty, Thomas went to examine Mr. Patel again as the nurse had reported he had been unwell in the night. This was the third time he had found Mr. Patel lying in a wet bed. He was very angry and went to tell the named nurse this was unacceptable and to change the bed. This left a bad atmosphere on the ward all day.

On reflection, Thomas realised that he probably had over-reacted, but it was because he felt so strongly about patients' dignity–he realised he had assumed that the nurses did not care as much as he did, but this was most likely not true, they were just really busy.

The next day, he went to apologise to the nurse. She thanked him and said she had felt really criticised but actually they had only just changed Mr. Patel, she was worried he was deteriorating and maybe he had a urine infection. They agreed to send off a sample and that they would talk more about how they could work better together in future.

---

This is an example of informal but purposeful reflection with Thomas being honest with himself and taking action to address unhelpful behaviours. Other types of reflection may involve written reflective accounts or a conversation with a colleague or supervisor and using a model or framework can help structure these and get the most out of the activity.

## Written reflection

All professionals are required to engage in written reflection at different stages of their training and career. This might be as part of a reflective portfolio (electronic or paper-based) or as part of formative or summative assessment. Written reflections can be structured using different models or frameworks, all of which involve some *description* of the event/situation; an *analysis* of what happened and how you felt and a *synthesis* which enables future *action*. This can be translated into one of the simplest models which is Borton's (1970) What? So What? Now What? Model.

Another framework for written reflections is Gibbs (1988) model:

Stage 1–Description of the event–what happened.
Stage 2–Thoughts and feelings (self-awareness).
Stage 3–Evaluation–what was bad or good about what happened.
Stage 4–Analysis–what did you and others do well, badly or not at all. In formal assessments, here is where you would include references from the literature or other evidence.
Stage 5–Conclusions–synthesise what you have discovered, what could you have done differently.
Stage 6–Action plan–what will you do next or differently?

### The professional conversation

Professional conversations may be structured around a significant event or case-based discussion as part of regular meetings with teachers, supervisors or colleagues. By encouraging story-telling, narrative and conversation in a structured way, the teacher can work with the learner to help them identify significant elements, learning points and areas for further reflection or development. The idea of 'developmental dialogue' is very common in educational activities such as peer review or observation, where experienced colleagues take the opportunity to engage in discussion around professional development. Defining outcomes, a structure, prompt questions and a time frame helps set clear boundaries around the conversation (McKimm, 2009).

## Feedback

Feedback can be defined as 'specific information about the comparison between . . . *observed performance and a standard, given with the intent to improve . . . performance*' (van de Ridder et al., 2008). Good feedback and professional conversations that stimulate reflection are essential for both learners and practitioners to develop their professional identities and learn from experiences. Good feedback needs to be:

• Authentic and constructive, for example *I felt you really connected with Mrs. Li Wing;*
• Timely, refer to specific examples and behaviours that can be changed, for example *you rushed through that history taking, you can take more time;*
• Tailored to the individual and their learning needs and stage;
• Aimed to encourage reflection through open questions, for example *did that go as you planned it? You will be talking with Mr. Jones' family tomorrow, how will you approach this in the light of what happened today?*

# 20 Ethics and the law

Learning outcomes:

- Understanding of what is meant by a professional code of conduct and how it relates to an ethical code
- Definitions of ethics, medical law, medical malpractice and medical negligence
- The similarities and differences in relation to personal and professional ethics
- Conscientious objection

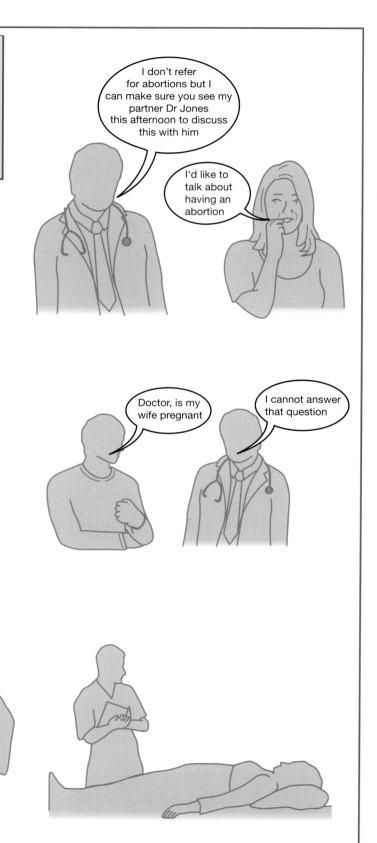

*Health Care Professionalism at a Glance*, First Edition. Jill Thistlethwaite and Judy McKimm.
© 2016 by John Wiley & Sons, Ltd. Published 2016 by John Wiley & Sons, Ltd.

# A professional code of conduct

One of the defining factors of a profession is that its members agree to adhere to a 'professional' code of conduct, which is derived in part from codes of ethics. A code of conduct governs and guides behaviour (how things should be done) and was originally an internal code defined and upheld within the profession itself. More recently in health care there have also been external influences on the code including lay and legal input. The original physician code is the Hippocratic oath, which many doctors still take on graduation in a updated format–they 'profess' the oath. In the United Kingdom, the GMC's *Good Medical Practice* stipulates the professional conduct of qualified doctors and there are similar publications in other countries.

Ethics and law applied to medicine and health care are included in most student programmes. Some courses begin with a theoretical introduction to the topics, whereas others focus very much on the practical implications. Remember that ethics is not only about big issues such as abortion, euthanasia and assisted suicide, but also about day-to-day issues such as confidentiality and open disclosure.

# Definitions

**Ethics** is the philosophical study of moral principles and rules to govern decision-making that then direct a person's actions. A code of ethics establishes whether and why an action is right or wrong. **Medical law** is the branch of law that focuses on the application of medical knowledge to legal issues.

**Medical malpractice** is 'any unjustified act or failure to act upon the part of a doctor or other health care worker which results in harm to the patient' (Kerridge et al., 2005).

Ethical practice is not synonymous with legal practice. We may all debate the ethics of particular cases and ethical dilemmas are common–there may not always be a consensus about what is right and what is wrong in a particular situation. However, what is legal or illegal is usually more obvious and is enshrined in law. Doctors, health professionals and students may receive advice about ethical issues from local ethics committees, and they may seek advice about legal problems from their professional defence bodies or their employing institution's legal department, for example.

## Personal versus professional ethics

Difficulties may arise when a health professional's personal values and ethical viewpoint are different from what is legal or illegal within the country in which she or he practises. An obvious example of this is when a doctor disagrees with abortion/termination of pregnancy on religious grounds yet abortion is legally allowed. The opposite may also be the case: before abortion was legalised in the United Kingdom, for example, many doctors performed terminations even though they were breaking the law.

**Conscientious objection** is an explicit legal right to freedom of thought, conscience and religion that may be limited in circumstances as defined by the law and in the interests of public safety, health or the protection of rights and freedoms of others.

> Consider other examples of where personal values and professional ethics may be at odds with what is legal or illegal; and then consider where you stand on such issues and how this may affect your work.

Health professionals have a right to conscientiously object to participating in management such as abortion, contraception and fertility treatment. However, they have to ensure that patients requesting such interventions are not disadvantaged and are referred to a practitioner who will take over their care.

Common ethical dilemmas occur when practitioners need to balance their duty of care to individual patients, families and society as a whole. Such dilemmas often involve confidentiality. For example, if a doctor tells a patient he is hepatitis B positive but the patient refuses to tell his wife and therefore puts her at risk of contracting the disease, the doctor may decide that the wife needs to be informed.

## Defining your ethical code

We live in a world of moral pluralism, the idea that there are few absolute rights and wrongs. This can lead to moral relativism: the view that ethical principles and morality are subject to a person's individual choice and that anything goes. However as a member of a profession, you are judged by your profession's code. As medical students you learn to think, to reflect and to debate in relation to ethics, as well as where to seek help and decide on the optimal course of action. Two important principles are beneficence (doing the right thing) and non-maleficence (doing no harm).

# Medical malpractice and negligence

Medical negligence results in harm to patients. The majority of malpractice claims relate to alleged negligence by a doctor. Patients or their families may subsequently sue for damages in court. Negligence may not be solely due to an individual doctor's behaviour but the system in which that doctor works. For negligence claims to be successful the prosecution must be able to show that the doctor involved had a duty of care to the patient, that the negligent action contributed to the patient's harm and that the doctor did not behave in a manner consistent with accepted medical opinion or standard care.

> Gita Mehta is a fourth-year medical student undertaking her obstetrics and gynaecology rotation in a university teaching hospital. Today she is in theatre for the gynaecology list with the professor operating. Gita is rather in awe of the professor who tells her to carry out a pelvic examination on the next patient, who has just been anaesthetised, in order to identify her ovarian cyst. What should Gita now ask before doing this internal examination?

Health professionals and students should always ask a patient for consent before carrying out any physical examination and they should explain what they are going to do and why. If consent is not requested and not received then this constitutes battery in many countries. The conduction of physical examinations by students on patients who are asleep without consent is thus battery. It is difficult for a student to query the instructions of someone senior. By learning about ethical and legal conduct students are made aware of what is permissible and hopefully the skills to question unethical behaviour.

# 21 Evidence-based practice

**Learning outcomes:**

- Definitions of evidence based practice (EBP)
- The nature and types of evidence
- The Cochrane Collaboration
- Formulating an answerable question-PICO

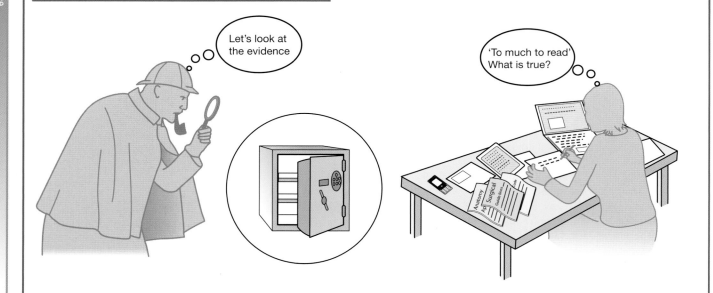

**The P.I.C.O. method of formulating a question**

**P** : identity the **population** or **patients** you are interested in
**I** : what is the management option, **intervention**, test etc. that you are considering?
**C** : is there an alternative to that intervention that serves as a **comparison**? (note there is not always a suitable comparator)
**O** : what is your preferred **outcome**? What do you hope to achieve or improve? The outcome should be measurable

Questions may be related to: medication/therapy/prevention; diagnosis, causation (aetiology), or prognosis.

Example: In men between the ages of 18 and 25 (P) is cognitive behavioural therapy (I) better than anti-depressants (C) for the treatment of mild depression (O)?

*Health Care Professionalism at a Glance*, First Edition. Jill Thistlethwaite and Judy McKimm.
© 2016 by John Wiley & Sons, Ltd. Published 2016 by John Wiley & Sons, Ltd.

# Why evidence-based practice

Evidence-based practice (EBP) (or evidence-based medicine, EBM) requires that all clinical decisions and management plans should have evidence to support them. At university you are learning how to search, appraise and apply evidence to clinical dilemmas and decision-making. You are also building up your knowledge base of evidence with the realization that not only will much of today's evidence be superseded by the time you are a practitioner but also that the available evidence may be flawed.

# Definition

'…the conscientious, explicit, and judicious use of current best evidence in making decisions about the care of individual patients. The practice of EBM means integrating individual clinical expertise with the best available external clinical evidence from systematic research. By individual clinical expertise we mean the proficiency and judgment that individual clinicians acquire through clinical experience and clinical practice…By best available external clinical evidence we mean clinically relevant research, often from the basic sciences of medicine, but especially from patient centred clinical research into the accuracy and precision of diagnostic tests…the power of prognostic markers, and the efficacy and safety of therapeutic, rehabilitative, and preventive regimens' (Sackett et al., 1996).

Note that evidence should be complemented by clinical judgement and experience.

# EBP 'in practice'

Newer, more powerful, accurate and effective tests and treatments often cost more than those they replace. The decision to implement new ways of working is made not only by individual professionals but also by health service managers and government departments. Everyone working in health care has a professional responsibility to be cost conscious.

> **Steps in EBP**
> 1. Convert information needs into answerable questions.
> 2. Track down the best evidence to answer these questions.
> 3. Critically appraise the evidence for its validity and importance.
> 4. Integrate this appraisal with clinical expertise and patient values to apply the results in clinical practice.
> 5. Evaluate performance.

# Where is the evidence?

Medical knowledge and health care are advancing so quickly that it is difficult to 'keep-up-to-date' with the evidence. There are more than 2000 articles published each week in over 20,000 journals. There will be a lot of reading and assimilation to fit around your service commitment as a doctor in training or other health care practitioner. Moreover, you must always keep-up-to-date and be a lifelong learner.

While we now have technologies to look up possible answers to clinical questions on the spot, it takes time to appraise what is often contradictory evidence from multiple sources and to decide which of those sources are credible. The easily accessible search engines such as Google and knowledge repositories such as Wikipedia are not always trustworthy. However, it is a useful exercise to search on symptoms and conditions through Google and look at the websites that patients are likely to be reading and ask for opinions on.

Research evidence adds to our knowledge. Knowledge translation is the exchange, synthesis and ethically sound application of that knowledge, within a complex system of interactions among researchers and users, to accelerate the capture of the benefits of research, that is, applying research results in clinical practice (Canadian Institutes of Health Research [CIHR], 2000). Doctors need to be able to search for evidence quickly when faced with unusual presentations or unfamiliar medication. The busy clinician running late in clinic or on a busy ward round is unlikely to find the time to search for, analyse and decide on the best answer to a clinical question. Providing as much synthesised information as possible, easily accessible, at the professional's desk or smart phone is absolutely necessary for EBP to translate into practice.

## The nature and types of evidence

The way in which evidence is generated through experimental data collection is categorised by 'strength of findings'. The double-blind randomised controlled trial (RCT) is seen as the gold standard in relation to drug efficacy. However, RCTs are expensive and pharmaceutical companies fund research raising questions of conflict of interest. Moreover, there has been a bias towards publishing positive results of trials and ignoring the ones that are equivocal or worse. It is therefore difficult to make judgements. Other types of quantitative evidence in decreasing order of quality are cohort studies, case studies, and expert opinion. Such evidence helps answer who, what, where and when questions. Qualitative evidence supplies richer and deeper data to explore why and how.

Health professionals sieve evidence to make decisions. Evidence comes from brief reading, conversations with peers, opinion leaders and pharmaceutical representatives, as well as your early training and experience. The 'trial of one' is a powerful decision aid: a doctor prescribes a new drug for the first time, the patient has an adverse reaction, and therefore the doctor is unlikely to prescribe that drug again, particularly if there are other well-tested options. Doctors also make diagnostic and treatment decisions based on the 'illness scripts' of patients they have seen in the past (Schmidt et al., 1990).

Systematic reviews do some of the work of evaluating evidence by analysing, criticising and synthesising all the published evidence on a particular topic employing strategies that limit bias and random error. Meta-analyses use statistical methods to combine the results of two or more quantitative studies. Qualitative reviews summarise research through a narrative approach.

## Systematic reviews: the Cochrane Collaboration

The Cochrane Collaboration is an international organisation that sifts medical evidence to produce systematic reviews across all specialties. Over 11,000 health professionals, researchers, scientists and consumers work in this area to answer clearly formulated questions of the type that clinicians ask every day in their work.

# 22 Values-based practice

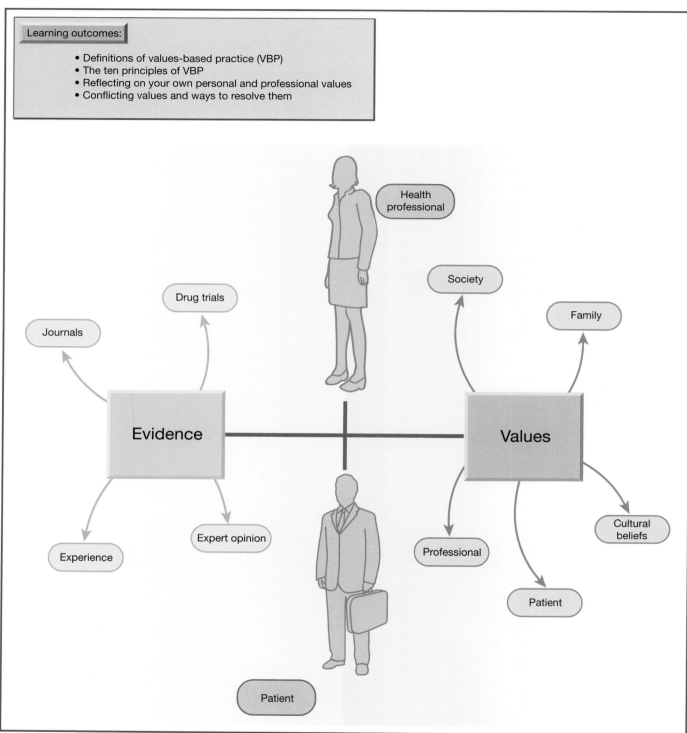

# Definitions

**Values** are 'the unique preferences, concerns and expectations each patient brings to a clinical encounter and which must be integrated into clinical decisions if they are to serve the patient' (Thornton 2006).

**Values-based practice** (VBP) is '. . . a blending of the values of both the service user and the health and social care professional, thus creating a true, as opposed to a tokenistic, partnership' (Thomas et al., 2010).

VBP links being patient-centred with the acknowledgment that health professionals' values affect interactions and the professional needs to be aware of these. VBP aims to involve both patient and doctor in decision-making and management, taking into account both parties' values and world views. It complements the EBP approach (Chapter 21). VBP is important as it helps health professionals understand the reasons why patients choose not to undertake a management plan as recommended, decline to take medicines as prescribed and are reluctant to modify their life styles. Doctors may present evidence which people choose to ignore, or the conclusions drawn from the evidence do not fit within patients' belief systems or resonate with their past experiences. A professional's choice and framing of evidence is similarly affected by their experience and values.

You need to be aware of and recognise differences in values and how these may affect your practice. Respect for values is a reciprocal process; the patient and all involved in care including the different professionals, carers and health services have to be aware of and respond to values, taking them into account in diagnosis, management and follow-up.

# What are your values?

> Consider what you mean by 'my values' and how they overlap with professionalism. Your values may be personal or professional. Do these differ? Have you ever been aware that your values differ from those of your friends, teachers and/or patients? What did you do/could you do in such circumstances?

You may refer to values as principles, beliefs, standards, a motivating force, your mission or even 'my conscience'. Sometimes we are not aware of our values until challenged, or put into a situation where others have different or opposing values, leading to potential conflict. Commonly held values are honesty, being fair, kindness, integrity, respect, obeying the law, working hard, helping people less fortunate than yourself, altruism, loyalty, self-reliance and putting others before yourself. Professional values may overlap with personal values: being punctual, not breaking confidentially and putting the patient first. Such values are fairly non-controversial. However, your value-system might also include a darker side: making sure you get your rights, aiming to be better than others (coming top of the class), doing whatever it takes to succeed and hanging out with influential people.

# Examples of conflicting values

> Jody is a medical student doing a medical rotation at the university teaching hospital. She is hoping to impress the senior physician who will grade the attachment with her work ethic and performance. The consultant asks her to present the history and examination of a patient she had seen that morning. Part way through she realises she did not take the patient's blood pressure. When asked for the reading she replies it was normal. Jody's desire to do well and not be 'told off' has conflicted with her value of honesty. She feels bad for the rest of the day.

> Peter is a nursing student working in general practice. He sees a patient with type 2 diabetes who has a body mass index of 36 and poor diabetic control. The patient says she is trying to lose weight. Peter is irritated as he feels that the patient is wasting health service resources by not taking control of her eating. He values self-control, exercising regularly to 'keep healthy'. He finds it hard to empathise with someone who obviously isn't trying hard enough to change. He does not explore the psychosocial circumstances of the patient and the reasons for her poor diet due to her low income.

# The ten principles of VBP

> **Practice skills**
> 1. Awareness
> 2. Reasoning
> 3. Knowledge
> 4. Communication
> **Models of service delivery**
> 5. User-centred
> 6. Multi-disciplinary
> **Values-based practice and evidence-based practice**
> 7. The 'two feet principle'
> 8. The 'squeaky wheel principle'
> 9. Science and values
> 10. Partnership
>
> (Fulford, 2004)

Health professionals need to consider the values in a given situation; this means not assuming what someone's values might be (either patients' or colleagues'). It is easy to make a value judgement about other people, and other professionals. In particular, we need to have an understanding about how our colleagues from other professions and disciplines might differ in their personal and professional values. Good communication helps prevent and resolve conflicts.

The 'two feet' principle is that all decisions are based on facts (evidence) and values. Can you think of instances where patients and professionals use different evidence bases because of their exposure to different media (journals, TV, Internet, etc.)? The 'squeaky wheel' principle is that values shouldn't just be noticed if there's a problem; exploring values early may prevent problems later.

# Values in practice

How do you ask other people about their values? VBP for consultations should be covered in your communication skills courses. Exploring your colleagues' values when working is more difficult. There may be opportunities to practise doing this if some of your education takes place with other health professional students; perhaps you will work in simulations together and consider professional values as part of the de-brief and feedback.

# 23 Cultural competency, sensitivity and safety

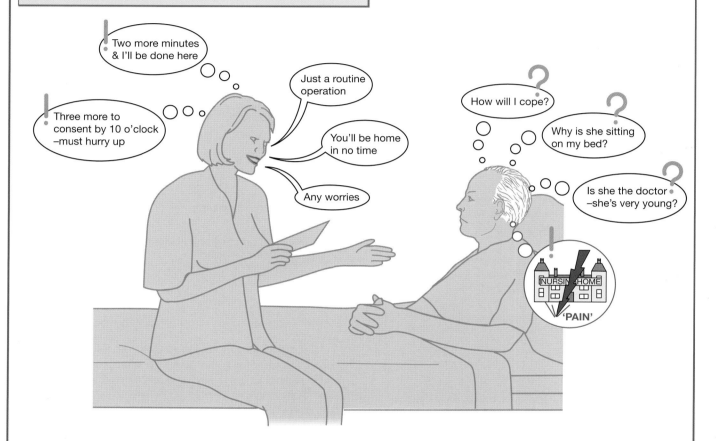

Culture influences peoples' health beliefs and 'illness narratives'. Instead of making assumptions, Kleinman and Benson (2006) suggest using an anthropological, ethnographic approach and using these questions to elicit individual's understanding of their illness:

–What do you call this problem?

–What do you believe is the cause of the problem?

–What course do you expect it to take? How serious is it?

–What do you think this problem does inside your body?

–How does it affect your body and your mind?

–What do you most fear about this condition?

–What do you most fear about the treatment?

*Health Care Professionalism at a Glance*, First Edition. Jill Thistlethwaite and Judy McKimm.
© 2016 by John Wiley & Sons, Ltd. Published 2016 by John Wiley & Sons, Ltd.

With ease of travel and migration patterns, health professionals work in increasingly diverse environments with individuals and communities from different cultural backgrounds. Whilst other social factors such as education, housing and poverty influence access to health care and health outcomes, structural inequalities and racism also play a part. Many interventions that aim to develop 'cultural awareness' focus on race and ethnicity. Although this is important, taking a broader view of what culture entails avoids possible stereotyping and includes taking account of gender, sexual orientation, socioeconomic status, faith, profession, tastes, disability, age, as well as race and ethnicity (Truong et al., 2014) and values (see Chapter 22).

## Definitions

*Culture* – the US National Institutes for Health (NIH) describes culture as 'the combination of a body of knowledge, a body of belief and a body of behavior. It involves a number of elements, including personal identification, language, thoughts, communications, actions, customs, beliefs, values, and institutions that are often specific to ethnic, racial, religious, geographic, or social groups. For the provider of health information or health care, these elements influence beliefs and belief systems surrounding health, healing, wellness, illness, disease, and delivery of health services' (http://www.nih.gov/clearcommunication/culturalcompetency.htm).

*Cultural competency* – the provision of services and care that are respectful of and responsive to the values; health beliefs; practices and cultural and linguistic needs of diverse patients, families and communities. It may require an adaptation of skills or approach to meet different patients' needs.

*Cultural sensitivity* – being aware that cultural differences and similarities exist and affect values, learning and behaviour.

*Cultural safety* – 'an environment that is spiritually, socially and emotionally safe, as well as physically safe for people; where there is no assault challenge or denial of their identity, of who they are and what they need. It is about shared respect, shared meaning, shared knowledge and experience of learning together' (Williams, 1999, p. 213). The concept was initially developed in New Zealand to support health care for the Māori people, but is useful for all health settings.

Being culturally competent involves reflecting and understanding how your own values, culture and beliefs influence the way they think and act; the care they provide and expectations about health, recovery, patients and families. This can be difficult as our own cultural influences are often taken for granted and not questioned.

- What do you think about these concepts?
- How might you put them into practice in your own work?
- How might you develop or enhance your own cultural competence and sensitivity?

## Cultural differences

Cruess and Cruess (2010) suggest that the way professionalism is defined should be tied closely to local, cultural and professional contexts. Cultural differences exist between Western models and other cultures which may focus less on the individual than the collective, and which often include a wider range of health workers, such as traditional healers or birth attendants as well as acknowledging the importance of spiritual aspects to well-being. For example, Al-Eraky et al.'s (2014) study in Arabian countries identified the 'Four-Gates' of medical professionalism: Dealing with Self, Dealing with Tasks, Dealing with Others and Dealing with God. The final gate includes two elements central to Arab culture, rooted in faith: self-accountability for own actions (taqwa) and self-motivation – expect reward from God, not people (ehtesab).

## Cultural competency in practice

So how do we put all this into practice?
- By reflecting honestly on our own culture, attitudes, beliefs and prejudices about 'others' (see Chapter 24)
- Demonstrating awareness and appreciation of and an open-minded attitude about others' beliefs and practices
- Promoting clear, value-free, open and respectful communication
  - Ask patients how they would like to be addressed
  - Become familiar with involving interpreters or translated written materials
  - Use simple, jargon-free, lay language (cancer instead of a tumour, heart attack instead of myocardial infarction, etc.)
- Developing trust – this may take more time especially if you are very different culturally from a patient or family
- Being prepared to involve other workers to meet patients' emotional, cultural and spiritual needs
- Recognising and avoiding stereotypical barriers
- Being prepared to engage with others in a two-way dialogue where knowledge is shared
- Not assuming anything, asking sensitive questions, being observant about verbal and non-verbal cues
- Treating people as individuals with their own identities and not as a representative of a group
- Understanding the influence of culture shock – including the culture of hospitals, clinics and medicine

Remember: what might seem simple, obvious or routine to you is probably unfamiliar, or even frightening, to patients or families.

# 24 Dealing with bias and prejudice

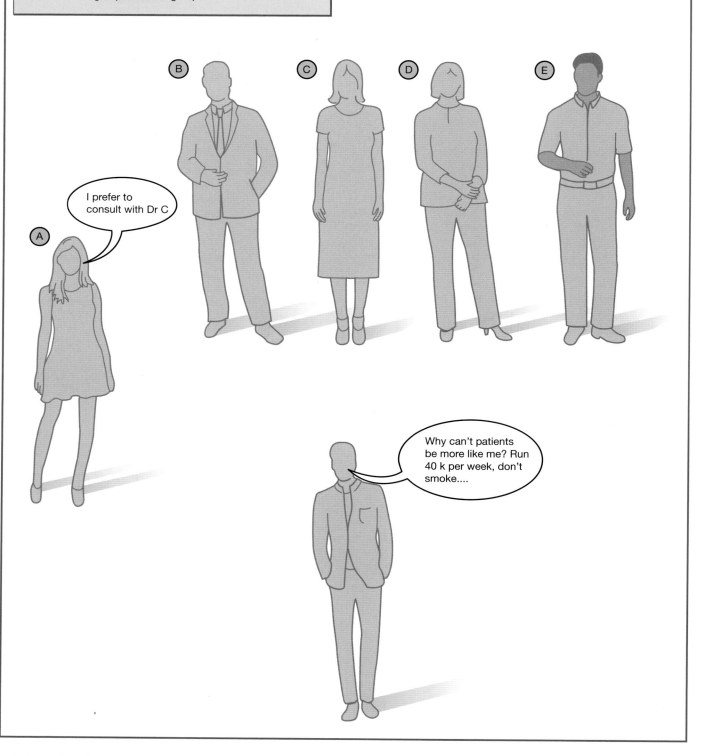

# Definitions

Bias and prejudice may be considered as synonyms, though they do have subtle differences in meaning. Bias is a preference that inhibits impartial judgement and is a word frequently used in statistics in a similar way: a statistical error caused by favouring certain outcomes over others. Bias can work both ways – a person, or test, can be biased for or against something. Prejudice, however, is an adverse judgment based on irrational negative bias or because of preconceived ideas and leads to an unfavourable outcome. Prejudice is commonly against someone with different opinions, characteristics or demographics compared to our own, for example because of gender, race, social class, sexuality or nationality.

There is no excuse for a health professional to display prejudice or to discriminate against anyone. However, we cannot judge people's attitudes towards others if they are not translated into observable behaviours including speaking and writing.

---

Consider your own biases and prejudices. What are they and why do you hold them – do you know? How might these affect your work as a health professional?
Now think of a time when you feel you have been the target of bias or prejudice. How did that feel? What can you learn from this experience in terms of your professional behaviour now and in the future?

---

# Preferences

Prejudice is different from a preference. For example, a female GP may prefer to consult with young and middle-aged female patients because she is able to empathise with this group and feels comfortable discussing women's health. She has a bias towards female patients but is not prejudiced against male patients; her patient satisfaction scores are similar across both genders and all ages.

In health care we try to respond to patients' preferences in relation to the gender of their health professional; but what other preferences should we agree to?

---

Duncan Perkins is a 70-year-old man attending the cardiology outpatient department. The clinic nurse calls him into the doctor's consulting room. Dr. Al-Eraky is of Middle Eastern appearance. Mr. Perkins loudly asks if he can see a white doctor, as he cannot understand 'them Asians'.
How should the doctor and nurse respond to this preference? Should the response be any different if the doctor were female and Mr. Perkins asked to see a male doctor instead?

---

# Prejudice in practice

People's prejudice arises from many sources. Our prejudices are connected to our values. One theory of prejudice suggests that it stems from four interlinked conditions (Stephan and Stephan, 1996):

- Negative stereotypes
- Intergroup anxiety
- Realistic threats (e.g. economic, physical)
- Symbolic cultural threats

## Negative stereotypes

We are all prone to stereotyping. Common examples are orthopaedic surgeons are poor communicators; unemployed teenagers are feckless and lazy; generation Y have poor attention spans; drug addicts are manipulative and cannot be trusted. Such stereotyping can affect how we relate to patients and we need to be on guard about how a patient looks and dresses, how they speak and whether they work affecting our professional behaviour.

## Intergroup anxiety

Humans normally feel more comfortable with people like themselves – their in-group. They may be suspicious and hostile towards member of other 'groups' – the out-group. An in-group is 'any cluster of people who can use the term "we" with the same significance' (Allport, 1979, p. 37). We would therefore refer to members of an out-group as 'they'. Of course, we may belong to several in-groups at any one time and over the course of our lives: as a health professional, as a medical professional, as a parent, as a football supporter, etc.

As professionals we may feel we don't understand certain groups of people or become frustrated because these groups don't understand and 'comply' with our professional advice. We feel anxious when interacting with people with different values and beliefs, and this leads to poor communication. We may move from wondering 'how can we help these people?' to 'they don't want our help so why should I bother?'

Intergroup anxiety may also cause difficulties between the professions. Medical students may stick together and not mix with nursing students, for example.

## Realistic threats

Realistic here is defined by the person with the prejudice. For example, we may define some people as misusing the health service particularly if we don't think they have contributed to the system through taxes or working. We act differently towards 'frequent attenders' or those we see as having trivial problems and therefore wasting our time.

## Symbolic/cultural threats

We may feel uneasy about the customs and behaviours of people from other cultures or belief systems. Examples are patients who decline blood transfusions on religious grounds; Muslim women in veils.

---

Parminder Singh is a third year nursing student on a placement in the Emergency Department. He is asked to talk to a heavily tattooed man of a similar age to himself. The patient admits he has been drinking heavily that afternoon – whisky and beer. He has also recently smoked some cannabis. He has fallen over and lacerated his face and hands. Parminder finds it hard to be 'professional' – he sees the guy as a total time waster who should get his act together and be responsible like himself. What type of people may you feel biased against and how might this affect your behaviour?

---

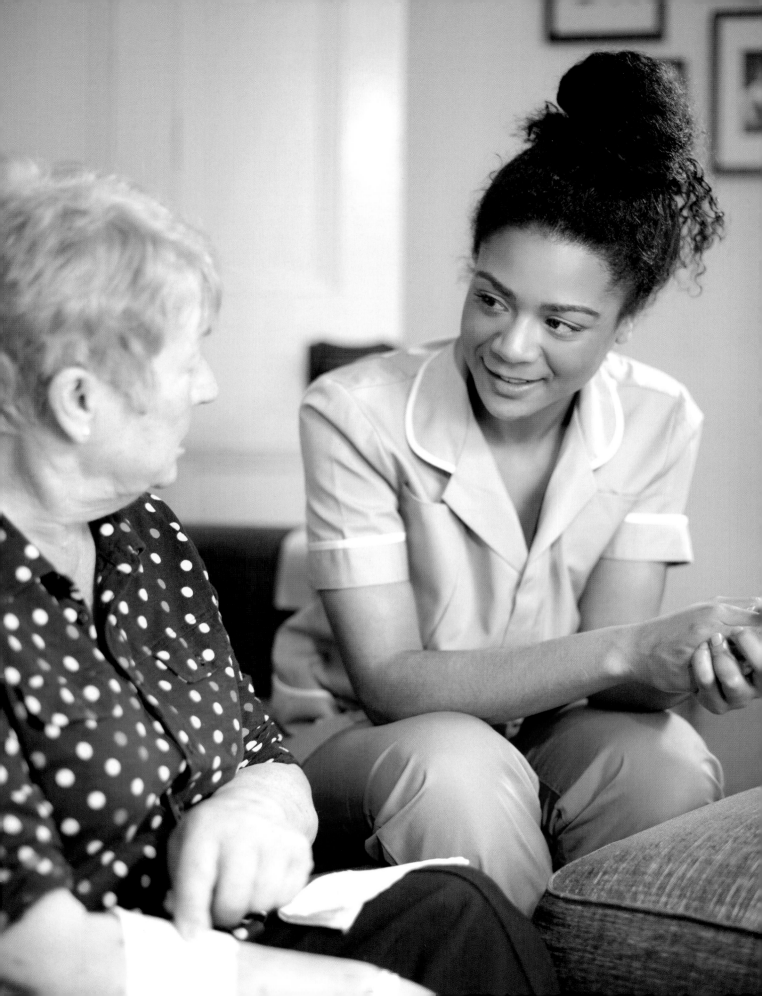

# Working with patients

## Part 4

## Chapters

# 25 Patient advocacy

## Menna Brown

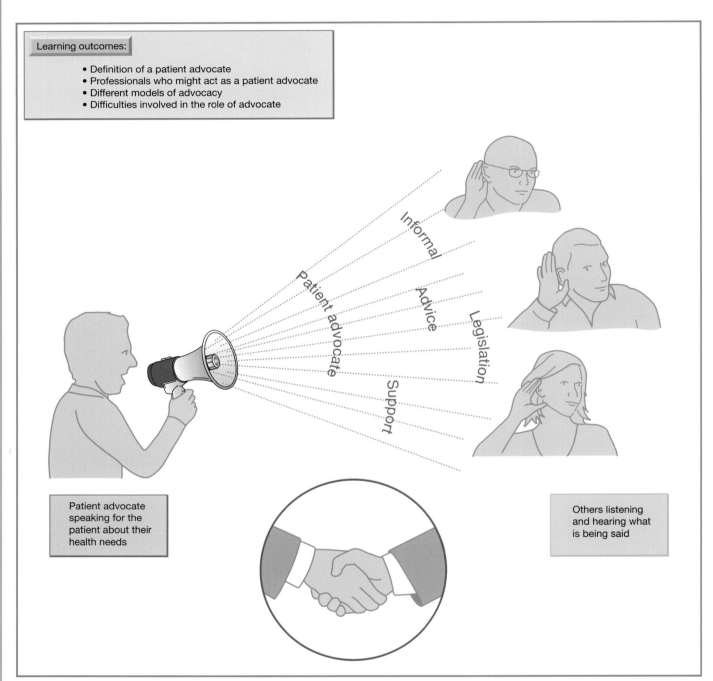

Learning outcomes:

- Definition of a patient advocate
- Professionals who might act as a patient advocate
- Different models of advocacy
- Difficulties involved in the role of advocate

Patient advocate
speaking for the
patient about their
health needs

Others listening
and hearing what
is being said

## Definition

There is no single definition of patient advocacy. The US National Patient Safety Foundation describes a patient advocate as a 'supporter, believer, sponsor, promoter, campaigner, backer, or spokesperson. . . . An effective advocate is someone you trust who is willing to act on your behalf as well as someone who can work well with other members of your healthcare team such as your doctors and nurses' (NPSA, 2003). It is important that patients and families have someone to advocate for them when they are unwell or under stress.

Advocacy comprises three essential components: valuing, apprising and interceding. All three are required to be present to realise

*Health Care Professionalism at a Glance*, First Edition. Jill Thistlethwaite and Judy McKimm.
© 2016 by John Wiley & Sons, Ltd. Published 2016 by John Wiley & Sons, Ltd.

'advocacy'. There are two specific antecedents of advocacy – a vulnerable population and the willingness to take responsibility for patient advocacy. The term has been linked to concepts of morality, ethics, autonomy, patient empowerment and self-determination.

## Patient Advocacy: Regulatory Framework

The Royal College of Physicians and Surgeons of Canada (CanMEDS) Framework (2005) has been integral to the development and understanding of patient advocacy across health care professions and has been replicated and utilised worldwide; it is being updated in 2015 through an extensive consultation process.

### Patient advocacy in medicine

The framework (2005) identified the role of patient advocacy within medicine; "The Role of Medical Expert is central to the function of physicians and draws on the competencies included in the Roles of Communicator, Collaborator, Manager, Health Advocate, Scholar and Professional". The advocate role encompasses individual patient care and extends it to include responsibility for the advancement of health and well-being of communities and populations.

### Patient advocacy in nursing

The International Code of Nursing (ICN) (1970) identified patient advocacy as a requirement of the nursing role; it later appeared in the Code of Professional Conduct (UK Central Council for Nursing, Midwifery and Health Visiting (UKCC), 1992) and within the Patients' Charter (1991) (DoH), which identified patients' right to certain expectations within their medical care and the right to complain if these were not met. Advocacy is found in all ethical codes for nursing, including the American Nurses Association (ANA) Code of Ethics for Nurses (2001) and is considered to have developed from increased confidence in nursing skills and professionalism.

Nurses have assumed the role of patient advocate, although all health professions have responsibilities to promote advocacy. Nurses are considered to be ideally positioned to act as patient advocates and, as members of a caring profession, able to actively promote it due partly to their proximity to and accessibility by patients. This enables them to discuss patient and family needs and bring issues to the attention of other professionals, including doctors. However, nurses are not legally acknowledged as patient advocates.

### Patient advocacy in pharmacy

The ASCP (2002) identified patient advocacy as a responsibility of pharmacists. As an accessible health professional, pharmacists are asked to take responsibility for the full medication process in order to enhance patient outcomes while acting as sources of information to aid patient access to community health resources and knowledge.

### The independent advocate

Professional independent advocate schemes exist which operate outside the health care system. Volunteers act to empower vulnerable groups, for example, older people or those with mental health issues. Professional advocates are free from conflicts of interest and other loyalties and are often trained explicitly to act as a patients' advocate.

### Family and friends as advocates

Family and friends are often in a unique position to be well informed of and understand patient's wishes. However, they may have a vested interest in patient outcomes and may misrepresent patients' needs as a result.

> How have you or could you act as a patient advocate? Are students able to take on these roles? Have you observed others acting on behalf of patients? Was this act supported by other health professionals?

## Models of Advocacy

Numerous models of patient advocacy exist. A philosophical view considers patients best placed to define their own best interest. Patient choice is the critical component, the advocate's role involves *assisting* the patient to interpret the situation and allow them to decide the best course of action. A pragmatic view focuses on self-determination and the role of the advocate to *inform* the patient and *support* them in their decision-making. This model assumes the ability of the patient to make an informed choice. Underpinning both these models is the assumption that individual advocates have the necessary skills and knowledge and empowerment to act as advocate (Dubler, 1992).

> Can you think of other ways to understand patient advocacy? Social workers are trained to advocate for those in their care. What could health professionals learn from this?

### Role of patient advocate

The role of patient advocate has been widely debated and there are arguments in support of the following:

- Create an atmosphere supportive of patients' decision-making
- Promote autonomy and informed consent
- Assist patients to find meaning in living or dying
- Promote and safeguard the interests of the patient
- Ensure patients have fair access to available resources
- Represent the views of the patient
- Educate and assist patient understanding of health care

## Barriers to patient advocacy

A number of potential barriers may limit an individual's ability to act as a patient advocate:

- Conflict of interest between responsibility to the patient and duty to employer
- Institutional constraints, lack of support, lack of power
- Lack of education and training for the role
- Limited continuity of care reducing ability to form caring bond with patient
- Traditional subservience to medical profession
- Potential personal consequences for advocating against the established system

> What other barriers may exist for health professionals involved in patient advocacy? Have you or your colleagues encountered any?

# 26 Patient Safety

## Menna Brown

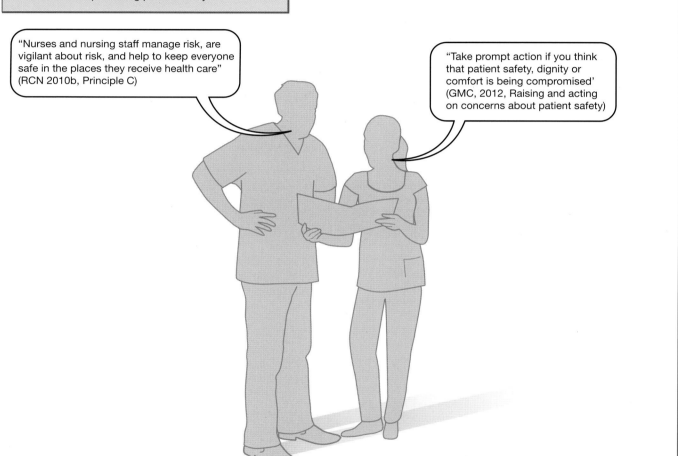

Learning outcomes:

- Definition of patient safety
- Global concerns and responses
- Role of health professionals in maintaining and promoting patient safety

"Nurses and nursing staff manage risk, are vigilant about risk, and help to keep everyone safe in the places they receive health care" (RCN 2010b, Principle C)

"Take prompt action if you think that patient safety, dignity or comfort is being compromised' (GMC, 2012, Raising and acting on concerns about patient safety)

*Health Care Professionalism at a Glance*, First Edition. Jill Thistlethwaite and Judy McKimm.
© 2016 by John Wiley & Sons, Ltd. Published 2016 by John Wiley & Sons, Ltd.

# Definition

**Patient safety** is the prevention of **errors** and **adverse effects** to patients associated with health care. It is also "the reduction of risks of unnecessary harm associated with healthcare to an acceptable minimum…the collective notions of given current knowledge resources available and the context in which healthcare was delivered weighed against the risk of non treatment or other treatment" (WHO, 2009). Moves to improve patient safety have gathered momentum over the last few decades, as a result of health improvement initiatives, generic concerns and major inquiries into mortality and morbidity rates, as well as the quality of health care and system errors.

# A global concern

Patient safety is a global concern with high incidence rates of errors and adverse effects reported across the world. Low resource countries are more at risk than high resource nations. In the European Union, data reported from member countries indicate that there is between an 8% and 12% occurrence rate for an 'adverse event', associated with hospital stays. Reported findings highlight the consistent nature of medical error across countries and associated patient safety issues.

The publication in 1999 of the US Institute of Medicine's (IOM) report 'To Err is Human: Building a safer health care system' brought a growing professional awareness for patient safety to the forefront of public minds. It marked the beginning of concerted efforts in the United States to tackle patient safety issues and address medical error which stood at more than 1 million injuries and 98,000 deaths annually.

Infections are reported to affect 4.1 million hospital patients a year; the four most common are urinary tract infection; lower respiratory tract infection; surgical site infection and MRSA (methicillin-resistant *Staphylococcus aureus*). Between 50% and 70% of medical errors could potentially be avoided through the adoption of a systematic approach to patient safety (WHO, 2009).

> Do you know what the annual infection rates are where you work/are on clinical placement and whether they are rising or falling? How do these compare to similar organisations?

# Global approaches

In 2002, the World Alliance for Patient Safety was formed consisting of 81 signatory countries representing 78% of the world's countries. The aim of the organisation is to produce a culture of patient safety, promote education and proactively identify risks. The first patient safety challenge was launched in October 2005 involving ministries of health from across the world with the aim of reducing healthcare associated infections (HAI) worldwide. Global experts from worked together to develop guidelines and toolkits to tackle issues concerning 'hand hygiene' and associated clean practices including the promotion of clean equipment, procedures, products, environments and water.

# System-wide strategies and solutions

In individual countries' health systems, the focus of health improvement is seen as everyone's business. Cultures are moving away from those of individual error, blame and punishment towards making system-wide and coordinated changes which work to defined protocols, procedures and proactive strategies, for example, the WHO Surgical checklist. In the United Kingdom, the National Patient Safety Agency (NPSA) was established to meet the challenges set by the WHO. (In 2012, its key responsibilities were transferred to the NHS Commissioning Board Special Health Authority.) NHS staff across the United Kingdom can report patient safety issues through confidential reporting locally or to the national reporting and learning system database. Data is collected and utilised to produce a range of patient safety resources including tool kits, checklists, alerts and feedback.

Following are the patient safety topics covered by NPSA (United Kingdom):

- Abuse/aggression and patient safety
- Consent, communication, confidentiality
- Documentation and patient safety
- Environment and patient safety
- Human factors and patient safety culture
- Medical devices/equipment
- Medication safety
- Patient accidents
- Patient admission, transfer, discharge
- Patient assessment and diagnosis
- Patient treatment and procedures
- Risk assessment and patient safety

# Health professionals' responsibilities

Whilst it is the core responsibility of every health professional to ensure they practise safely on a day-to-day basis, engagement at system level with safety concerns is also a core professional behaviour. Coordinated, formalised quality improvement, clinical governance, audit and monitoring processes are now well embedded in many organisations. Involvement in data gathering, reporting and follow-up is therefore a key role of most health professionals. Following clinical protocols and procedures and identifying risks are also seen as critical. Guidance and codes of practice on patient safety and expectations for all health professions are clearly set out and whilst certain groups have key-defined responsibilities (such as pharmacists being responsible for the safe provision of medication), many different health professionals are involved in the chain of activities that lead to a patient taking prescribed drugs safely and appropriately.

> Many formal reports on substandard health care identify that poor communication and coordination between groups, departments and organisations is a critical component. Taking one of the topics listed above, can you identify a situation in which an error, adverse event or near miss occurred recently? Why do you think this happened; how do you think this could have been prevented?

# 27 Relationships with patients

**Learning outcomes:**

- The nature of relationships
- Understanding the implications of physical touch in clinical settings
- Professional power and relationships
- The use of chaperones

*'Whatever houses I may visit, I will come for the benefit of the sick, remaining free of all intentional injustice, of all mischief and in particular of sexual relations with both female and male persons, be they free of slaves'*
Edelstein L. (1943). *The Hippocratic Oath. Text. Translation and interpretation.* Baltimore: John Hopkins Press.

**Chaperones**

Under what circumstances should you think about having a chaperone when you interact with patients? Does this depend on your gender? The patient's gender? The patient's age?

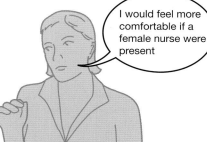

*Health Care Professionalism at a Glance*, First Edition. Jill Thistlethwaite and Judy McKimm.
© 2016 by John Wiley & Sons, Ltd. Published 2016 by John Wiley & Sons, Ltd.

# No intimate relationships

Everyone knows that doctors are not allowed to have intimate relationships with their patients. Or to put it more plainly – you should not have sex with a patient. However there is more than sex to consider about professional relationships with patients.

The General Medical Council (GMC, 2013c) states 'You must not use your professional position to pursue a sexual or improper emotional relationship with a patient of or someone close to them'.

The quotes highlight the enormous trust that people place in their doctors; they invite health professionals into their homes and, when sick enough to merit a home visit, patients are often at their most vulnerable. While home visits are not as common these days, doctors are often still in a position to abuse the trust of their patients when performing physical examinations. Less commonly, doctors are also at risk from patients who make inappropriate advances or accuse doctors of inappropriate behaviour.

## Physical touch and the clinical environment

> Have you ever considered the unusual degree of intimacy that you are granted/will be granted when examining patients? From simply taking a pulse, to palpating an abdomen, to examining breasts…

Patient–doctor interactions should take place in a neutral environment to promote trust and confidentiality. However, it is often difficult to find such a neutral environment. The hospital ward and the doctor's surgery are clinical environments where doctors are more at ease than worried patients. GPs in particular, who may practise in the same space for many years, have to consider whether their room should be 'clinical', and potentially off-putting for some, or warm and welcoming with muted colours and artwork.

> How would you furnish your medical office to balance the need for detachment and warmth? Think of clinical environments you have been in – what do you prefer in terms of décor? Would you have photographs of your family displayed or do you consider that unprofessional? Why?

You may have noticed different lay-outs of consulting rooms. For example, there is usually a great deal of thought put into the relationship of the desk and chairs, and the position of the computer if present. Many doctors no longer sit across a desk from their patients but arrange the seating so that there is no barrier between them, just perhaps the corner of a table. The aim is to try to bridge the power gap between the patient and professional. This has also meant shedding the white coat in some cases, though it is also disappearing in hospitals to reduce the spread of infection.

## Former patients, power and protection

The GMC's guidance also advises caution in relation to former patients. It does not suggest there should be a complete ban on sexual relationships. There are exceptions to most rules but the GMC's aim is to protect vulnerable people. In certain locations it may be difficult to avoid former patients entirely. For example in rural and remote areas of Australia and Canada there may only be one or two doctors practising. Single doctors marrying locals helps retain the professional in an area of need. 'Falling in love' with mutual consent is unlikely to lead to a complaint. However, you do need to consider the nature of the former patient's problem. It may be defined as unethical if the patient had a mental health problem and you were involved in giving counselling or psychotropic medication.

So the underlying issue is the power imbalance inherent in patient–doctor relationships and the possible long-term adverse consequences for patients. They may develop problems such as depression, anxiety disorders, psychosexual dysfunction, inability to trust health professionals in future encounters, guilt and feelings of worthlessness, as well as increased drug and alcohol use.

---

**Examples of sexual misconduct**
- Conducting examinations without permission (e.g. while patient is anaesthetised or unconscious): the patient needs to give consent. You should not carry out such an examination even if asked by someone senior without establishing that such consent has been obtained. The examinations do not need to be intimate.
- Rendering a patient into such a state that he/she is unable to refuse intimacy (e.g. giving patient drugs, hypnosis).
- Conducting physical examinations that are unnecessary in relation to the history/possible diagnosis such as pelvic or breast. Always explain why you are carrying out an examination and use a chaperone as appropriate.
- Frotteurism (achieving sexual stimulation or orgasm by touching and rubbing against a patient).
- Watching patients undressing or dressing.
- Using overt sexual language that is inappropriate.

---

## Chaperones

Having a chaperone present protects both the patient and the doctor. Doctors may be accused falsely of sexual harassment and even assault. The NHS Clinical Governance Support Team published a model chaperone framework in 2007. It states 'for most patients respect, explanation, consent and privacy take precedence over the need for a chaperone. The presence of a third party does not negate the need for adequate explanation and courtesy and cannot provide full assurance that the procedure or examination is conducted appropriately' (p. 3). The Royal College of Obstetricians and Gynaecologists recommends that patients having intimate examinations should be offered a chaperone irrespective of the gender of the doctor or nurse and that if the patient declines this request should be honoured and noted in the medical records. Doctors may be accused of unprofessional conduct if they do not have a chaperone present. Unprofessional behaviour also includes overexposure of the patient's body, inappropriate comments, inappropriate gestures or body language and putting the patient in an unorthodox position.

# 28 The nature of autonomy: patient and doctor

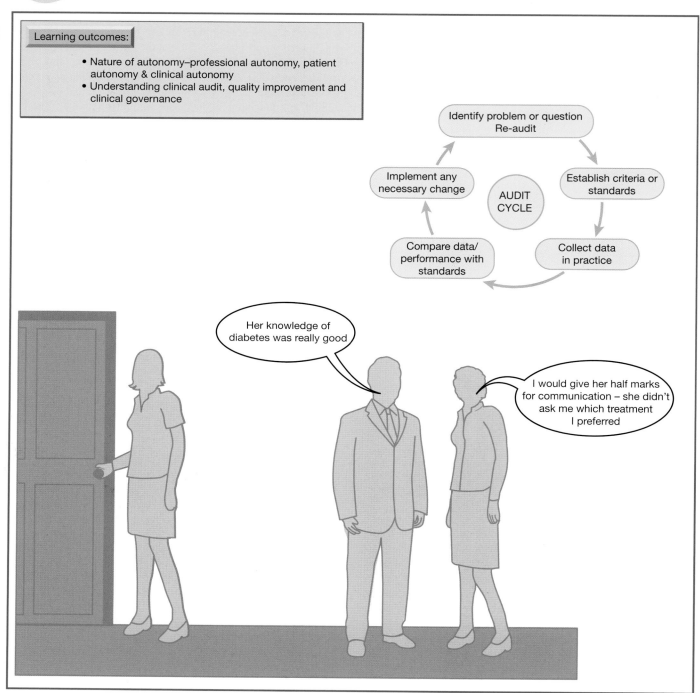

Learning outcomes:

- Nature of autonomy–professional autonomy, patient autonomy & clinical autonomy
- Understanding clinical audit, quality improvement and clinical governance

Identify problem or question
Re-audit

Implement any necessary change

AUDIT CYCLE

Establish criteria or standards

Compare data/ performance with standards

Collect data in practice

Her knowledge of diabetes was really good

I would give her half marks for communication – she didn't ask me which treatment I preferred

## Definition

Autonomy is the right of self-government – though in the case of the professions this usually means the right to self-regulation.

> Consider the similarities and differences between professional autonomy and the more recent concept of patient autonomy. Are there any conflicts between the two?

## Professional autonomy

The justice system in many countries includes the right for a person to be judged by one's peers, that is one's equals. So the professions consider it is important that their members are judged by colleagues from the same profession. This usually means judged in terms of suitability to practise and to continue to practise that profession. Remember that the definition of profession includes there being a unique and complex body of knowledge and skills that members learn and possess. Therefore logically only members can assess other members as no one from outside the profession has the capability to do so. Medical students are assessed primarily by doctors, who set the questions and decide whether to pass or fail the examinees at OSCEs, long cases and so on. For many years it was also doctors who decided whether another doctor should be allowed to stay on the medical register after any transgressions or questions about unprofessional conduct.

In recent years the medical profession has lost some of this autonomy. Some would say this has eroded the medical profession's status whereas others consider that the general population should have a say in who is allowed to provide health care.

Autonomy is a complex concept and is not simply about who has the power to remonstrate with a doctor, apply conditions to how and where a doctor works, or remove a doctor's name from the medical register. In the United Kingdom, within the National Health Service, the state, in negotiation with the profession, sets the terms of service and the remuneration for public doctors. British doctors have never been wholly free from state control. More recently doctors have seen restrictions put on public prescribing and referrals to secondary care. Their ability to make decisions based solely on clinical need has been eroded.

## Patient autonomy

Patient autonomy, patient partnership, patient safety, consumerism and charters have affected how medicine is practised. *The Patient's Charter* (Department of Health, 1991, revised editions in 1995 and 1997) defined the rights of patients and the standards of service they should expect within the NHS.

On the whole patients **trust** their doctors. They do not want the state interfering in doctors' decision-making though many want their own opinions heard in terms of treatment. If patients feel that the government is putting pressure on doctors' clinical decisions that trust may be eroded.

## Changes affecting professional autonomy

- Introduction of mandatory clinical audit and governance
- Clinical standards defined
- Revalidation to ensure clinical competence maintained
- Framework for assessing professional performance
- Definition of responsibility within team-based care
- Research into complex systems and how they succeed or fail
- Better system of informed consent
- Measures to improve communication skills of doctors particularly in relation to discussion of risk
- Importance of patient safety stressed and measures to ensure this
- Stressing of the importance of doctors monitoring their colleagues' clinical activity and taking prompt action once problems diagnosed

The GMC now includes 14 lay members together with 19 doctors elected by their peers and two academics representing the royal colleges and the universities. Some medical schools include patients in their assessment processes – for example patients mark students on their communication in OSCEs. Patients, of course, have for some time been involved in giving formative feedback to students – either as simulated patients or 'real' patients.

> What are you views on involving patients in decisions about medical students' and doctors' performance? Have you experience of being assessed by a patient? What effect has patient feedback had for you?

## Clinical autonomy

Clinical autonomy is the freedom of doctors to define the needs of their patients and to use state/health service resources to meet those needs (Alaszewski, 1995). Clinical audit and clinical governance are now important exercises within the NHS and doctors have to show evidence of audit activity in their annual appraisals and revalidation process. The purpose of audit is to improve the quality of service and clinical delivery to patients and to enhance cost effectiveness and efficiency, at the expense of complete clinical autonomy.

> **'Clinical audit is a quality improvement process** that seeks to improve patient care and outcomes through systematic review of care against explicit criteria and the implementation of change. Aspects of the structure, processes and outcomes of care are selected and systematically evaluated against explicit criteria. Where indicated, changes are implemented at an individual, team or service level and further monitoring is used to confirm improvements in health care delivery.' (NICE, 2002)
> **Clinical governance** is a system through which NHS organisations are accountable for continuously improving the quality of their services and safeguarding high standards of care by creating an environment in which excellence in clinical care will flourish.
> **Quality improvement** is about making health care safer, effective, patient centred, timely, efficient and equitable.

# 29 Boundary crossings and violations

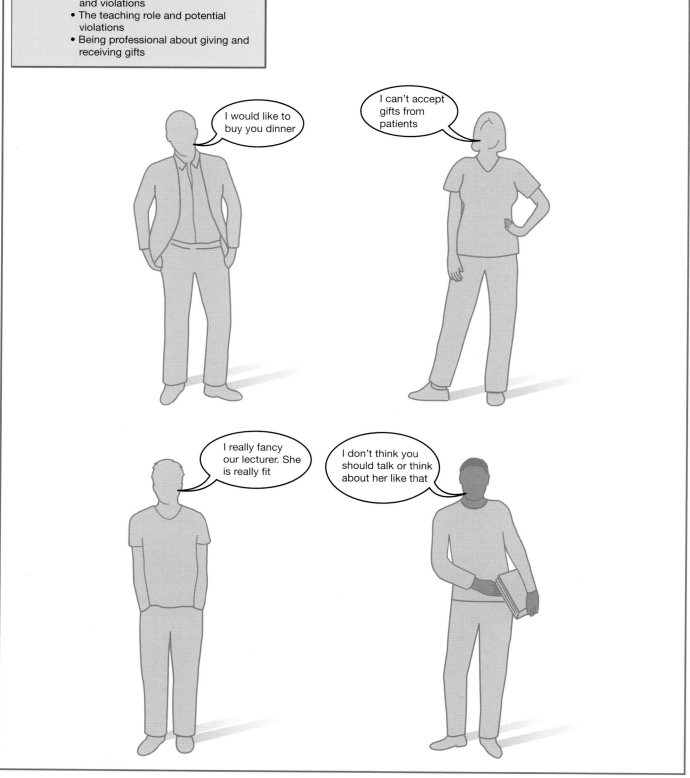

*Health Care Professionalism at a Glance*, First Edition. Jill Thistlethwaite and Judy McKimm.
© 2016 by John Wiley & Sons, Ltd. Published 2016 by John Wiley & Sons, Ltd.

# Definitions

Boundary violations occur when a patient, or a professional, acts in such a way as to satisfy non-therapeutic desires or goals in what should be a therapeutic relationship. There is a difference between a boundary crossing and a violation. The former is not exploitative and may be helpful to patients, but violations are always harmful (Galletly, 2004). Boundary crossings can lead to violations – sexual relationships often develop after a series of boundary crossings (Galletly, 2004). Violations arise from the power imbalance in relationships – professionals have power in consultations even if they may not always be aware of this on a day-to-day basis.

> In what ways may this power imbalance affect patient–doctor relationships?

## Boundary crossings

Boundary crossings may start when a health professional tries to bring an interaction with a patient onto a more even level, negating the perceived power imbalance. Patients and professionals may use first name terms. Clinicians may divulge information about their own lives or have photographs of their family on their desk. A relaxed style may help patients feel comfortable in discussing their problems. However, such behaviour may also cause a vulnerable patient to believe that the relationship has a life and meaning outside the consulting room, which the professional never intended to convey.

## Boundary violations

Boundary violations may also occur if a professional tries to impose his or her own values onto a patient: these may be religious, political and/or moral. For example, in 2010, a patient complained to the GMC about a consultation in which he said that the doctor spoke to him about religion. The doctor was alleged to have said that faith in Christianity would help the patient overcome his personal problems.

---

**Warning – boundary violation**
- Seeking a patient's company outside the consulting room/hospital
- Telling patients personal/intimate details about yourself
- Accepting presents from patients
- Giving presents to patients
- Thinking that a patient's life would be better if he/she has sex with you
- Feeling excited before the patient's next appointment
- Daydreaming about a patient
- Feeling let down if a patient consults another doctor or health professional
- Enjoying feeling that you have power over a patient
- Asking patients to do personal favours for you like posting a letter
- Making special arrangements for a patient such as seeing them after surgery hours

---

# Violating the teaching role

Boundary crossings and violations may also occur outside your clinical roles and settings. You will certainly be aware from the media of the responsibilities of school teachers towards their pupils and the need for teachers to maintain an appropriate professional distance. OK – at university you and your teachers are adults but is it acceptable for a tutor/teacher and students to

- Give and receive additional one-to-one coaching?
- Attend social events together outside the university?
- Buy each other drinks?
- Give each other presents?
- Have an affair?

Students certainly will be attracted to their colleagues; student doctors go out with other health professional students and with qualified nurses and other graduates. But what do you feel about a relationship between the consultant whose team you are attached to and a student in your year group? Is this exploitative? Does it make any difference in terms of gender? Is it professional?

Certainly if the couple try to keep the relationship a secret, they must feel guilty or embarrassed in some way. Boundary violations may also be fiduciary, that is, the student gives favours to the teacher for financial or academic gain. For example, teachers may award higher grades or write glowing references for favours rendered that do not accurately reflect the student's actual performance.

### Giving and receiving gifts

---

Mrs. Trudy Bowler is being discharged from hospital today after a major operation from which she has made a full recovery. She says goodbye to the nurses and gives them two large boxes of chocolates. As a senior student you have seen Mrs. Bowler most days for the last 3 weeks and always made a point of checking on her progress and encouraging her to mobilise. On that last day she hands you an envelope. It contains £200 and a thank you note.

---

Patients should never be encouraged to give gifts. The GMC advice for doctors is that 'You must not ask for or accept – from patients, colleagues or others – any inducement, gift or hospitality that may affect or be seen to affect the way you prescribe for, treat or refer patients or commission services for patients. You must not offer these inducements' (GMC, 2013a). But there are no guidelines about what you should do about presents given without solicitation. Mrs. Bowler may be offended if you decline her gift. Hopefully she knows you are a student so does not think that you will give her enhanced medical benefits in the future. Are the issues the same whether you are a student, doctor in training or fully qualified? What should you do about this gift?

Professional behaviour should mean your reflecting on the gift, its cost, its meaning and implications of accepting or rejecting it. Students and junior health professionals who are given presents should seek advice from a senior member of staff. Monetary gifts could be donated to charity and the patient advised. Certainly tax payers need to declare such gifts as income.

# 30 Compliance, adherence and shared decision-making

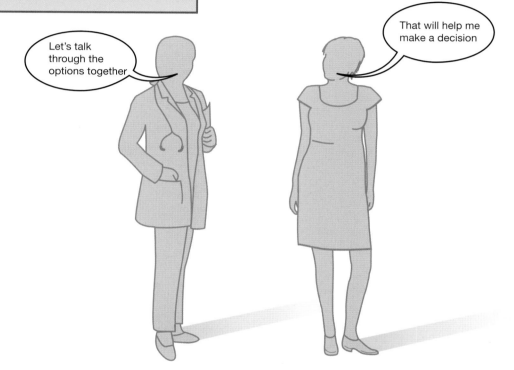

Learning outcomes:

- Why you should avoid the use of the word 'compliance'
- The nature of and skills for shared decision making with patients
- What information patients would like when making decisions
- How value judgements affect choices

Let's talk through the options together

That will help me make a decision

**Health Literacy** refers to the cognitive and social skills that influence the motivation and ability of people to gain assess to understand and than make use of information to promote and maintain good health, and to help prevent poor health and illness.

**While Health Literacy** includes the ability to read health information leaflets, make appointments with health care professionals and navigate the health service, it also implies enhancing a person's access to information and their capability to use and act on that information.

Adapted from: The World Health Organization's track 2-health literacy and health behaviour
Available at:

http://www.who.int/healthpromotion/conferences/7gehp/track2/en/

## Not compliance

Have you heard the statement: 'the patient is not compliant'? What does this indicate in terms of being patient-centred? It usually translates as 'the patient is not doing what the doctors have ordered'. A compliant patient is a passive patient. The doctor who prefers compliant patients is usually practising in a paternalistic manner.

## But involvement

These days most patients want to be involved in decisions about their care and the care of their families – 'no decision about me, without me'. They will **adhere** to management plans if they receive enough information about their problem, understand the meaning of their condition and the options available, and are able to enter into a dialogue with the health professional about the treatment. Therefore, they are not passive but take an active role in their own management. After all – the patient is the person who decides whether to swallow their prescribed pills or to stop smoking. This shared decision-making approach is a feature of the **therapeutic relationship** and patient-centred practice and requires excellent communication including negotiation skills. The **health literacy** of the patient also needs to be taken into account.

> A therapeutic relationship occurs between a patient and a professional: it is safe, reliable, confidential and appropriate.

As noted in Chapter 32, skills you need to learn and practise are the ability to translate medical terminology (or jargon) into understandable language, and to check that understanding without being patronising or making assumptions about a patient's prior knowledge. What words and terms you use will depend on the patient's experience, their occupation, educational attainment, age and/or cultural background. However, such judgements may be flawed due to your own values and stereotyping. Patients may need explanations about investigations, how procedures are performed, how a particular disease or condition may affect them, long-term effects of the condition or treatment, the prognosis, what treatment options are available, their side effects and so on.

> **Information needs of patients (from Coulter et al., 1999)**
> • Understanding what is wrong
> • A realistic idea of prognosis
> • The processes and likely outcomes of possible tests and treatments
> • How to assist in self care
> • Available services and sources of help
> • Reassurance and help to cope
> • Helping others understand
> • Legitimising seeking help and their concerns
> • How to prevent further illness
> • How to identify further information and self-help groups

### Shared decision-making

Shared decision-making is more likely to happen when there are several options, each of which has advantages and disadvantages.

Health professionals have a certain amount of power as to which options are described. They may also influence the patient's choice by the amount of information given about each option; patients may pick up on a doctor's preference, for example, which affects their choices. A positive outcome is when both the patient and the practitioner finish an interaction feeling satisfied with the outcome. Both may then consider that the practitioner has acted professionally.

> Dr. Edward Jones is discussing a management plan for the treatment of Susan Smith's morbid obesity. There are several options available all of which have different advantages and disadvantages. One of the better options is only available at a substantial cost to patients. Dr. Jones does not mention this choice as he feels Susan would not want to pay for the treatment. Is Dr. Jones acting professionally? What would you do in this situation? What might Susan prefer?

Professionalism issues here are when professionals are influenced by personal gain in terms of management – for example if a doctor has a financial stake in a pathology laboratory or has been promised inducements by pharmaceutical companies.

## Value judgements and choice

We need to be careful about making value judgements about patients' choices – what we think they may or may not want to hear, and what we think their best options are (see Chapter 22). By asking about a patient's ideas, concerns and expectations (the 'ICE model'), doctors can begin to gauge a patient's possible choice but need to check that they have shared the decision-making process. Of course, the doctor as expert in the management of the condition should present the pros and cons of the options; the doctor then facilitates the patient's decision recognising the patient as an expert on his/her condition. A patient may ask 'what would you do doctor'? The doctor may give a preference but relate this choice to the patient's situation and explain that it may not be the best option for that situation.

Patients expect their doctors and health professionals to present information in a way they can understand. Research has shown that how information is presented is more important than the amount (Wright et al., 2004). Patients on the whole trust their health professionals and expect their questions to be answered honestly.

Frequently patients and practitioners share a decision to do nothing. So they adopt a 'wait and see' option, which means dealing with some uncertainty. Continuity is important here and the patient needs to be advised what to watch out for in terms of deteriorating symptoms. Being able to cope with uncertainty is important for health professionals.

Of course, patients may want to have investigations for what a doctor feels is a self-limiting problem. This situation involves a lot of negotiation and reassurance. Some symptoms are just part of normal human experience (e.g. not sleeping after the break-up of a relationship) and do not necessarily mean illness. The process of recognising that symptoms are not pathological is 'normalisation' (Kessler and Hamilton, 2004).

# 31 Prescribing: medication and management

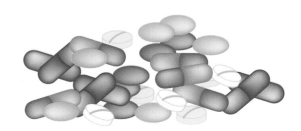

- The importance of getting prescribing right
- Patient safety implications of prescribing errors
- Information needs of patients in relation to drugs

**Prescription requirements:**

Patient's name and address

Name of medication, strength and dosage
Special instructions on how to take
(eg with food, with plenty of water, at night etc)

Number/amount to be dispensed

Prescriber's signature
Name of prescriber
Prescriber's number or other form of identification
depending on country
Date

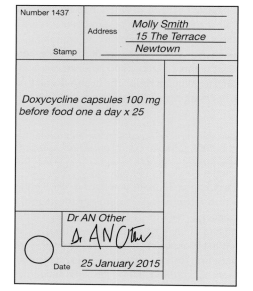

| Number 1437 | Stamp | Address | Molly Smith
15 The Terrace
Newtown |

Doxycycline capsules 100 mg
before food one a day x 25

Dr AN Other

Dr AN Other

Date 25 January 2015

# Becoming a prescriber

Surveys of newly qualified doctors in training consistently include data that show that graduates lack confidence in prescribing. There are many possible explanations for this deficit in what is a key area of professional practice. Obviously medical students are not legally allowed to prescribe for patients and therefore they may have infrequent opportunities to practise prescribing. They may be asked to suggest management plans for patients but not actually write the plan down. The drug charts and prescription pads that require completion may be mystery objects whose importance only becomes apparent on the first day of work. A data sheet contains information on a drug's indications for use, mode of action, dose, risk profile, interactions, use in pregnancy, the aged and children, and necessary monitoring. These are available online and versions for patients and prescribers are included in a drug's packaging.

To remedy this obvious deficit the United Kingdom has introduced the PSA – prescribing skills assessment – that each final year medical student needs to pass before being allowed to start work after graduation. This is a national assessment and not part of a medical school's examination menu (www.prescribe.ac.uk/psa/).

As students you may be able to administer medicines and injections under supervision. Do not do this if you feel uncomfortable and ensure that you have the correct training with feedback.

## Patient safety and prescribing errors

Mistakes when prescribing are a major source of patient safety problems. Errors occur for many reasons including the individual prescriber, the environment in which prescribing takes place and organisational factors. There may be lack of knowledge, suboptimal training, poor supervision, excessive workload, tiredness and insufficient checking of junior staff. Many adverse drug reactions are avoidable and are commonly due to not recording and/or checking a patient's allergies, giving the wrong dosage, inappropriate route of administration, drug interactions and existing medical conditions. Estimates of the health burden from adverse drug reactions vary but figures commonly quoted are: 2–3% of hospital admissions are related to drug events (Roughead and Semple, 2009); 28% of patients attending emergency departments in the United States have a drug-related problem or inappropriate prescription with 70% of these preventable (Patel and Zed, 2002); 7.5% of prescriptions in ambulatory settings have errors in Europe (European Medicines Agency – www.ema.europa.eu/ema/).

## Prevention of adverse drug events:

- Ensure you have selected the appropriate medication and dosage, including frequency and route of administration, for the correct patient (check patient records, patient identity and confirm with patient/carer).
- Check for allergies, previous drug-related problems, etc.
- Look up information if necessary rather than relying on memory for drug dosage and risk profile.
- Minimise polypharmacy (multiple prescriptions for the same patient).

- Write or preferably print legible prescriptions
- Sign and date prescriptions.
- Record prescription in the patient record/chart.
- Check patient understanding of prescription.
- Use Dosette boxes if appropriate in the community.
- Remember the role of the pharmacist (hospital or community) and ask for advice as appropriate.

## Reporting systems

Of course not all adverse events are due to error. In particular reactions to new drugs are unpredictable. Highly controlled drug trials before mass marketing will not necessarily show up all the possible effects of a medication and therefore new events will occur that are not listed in the drug data sheet. In many countries health professionals are required by law to report adverse drug events that are not already listed in the drug profile. These events can then be investigated, monitored and researched further. Eventually the drug data sheet will be updated or, in some cases, the drug may be withdrawn from availability.

The system in the United Kingdom is called the 'yellow card system' and is run by the MHRA (Medicines and Healthcare products Regulatory Agency) and the Commission on Human Medicine (https://yellowcard.mhra.gov.uk). Patients are also encouraged to report problems, particularly for over-the-counter medications and cosmetic treatments. In Australia, the Advisory Committee on the Safety of Medicines (ACSOM – www.tga.gov.au/about/committees-acsom.htm) monitors drug events and these are then published in the *Australian Prescriber* (www.australianprescriber.com/). In the United States, the main reporting centre is operated by the Food and Drug Administration (FDA).

# Patient information needs

As a prescriber it is also very important to include patients in decisions about medications, particularly those we expect them to take regularly, as we saw in chapter 30. Research has shown that patients have four particular information needs in relation to new medication (Dickinson and Raynor, 2003):

**Essential information patients want about drugs**
- What it does and what it's for
- Side effects (possible and common)
- Do's and don'ts (can I take other medication with it?)
- How to take it (how often, when, with food?, chew or swallow, etc.)

Patient advice leaflets in drug packets are now much easier to understand and it is good practice to advise patients to read these and ask questions if necessary – of the pharmacist particularly.

# Other prescribers

In some countries other health professionals as well as doctors may prescribe after appropriate training; for example, in the United Kingdom nurse practitioners, pharmacists and dentists have this right within certain limits.

# 32 Communication

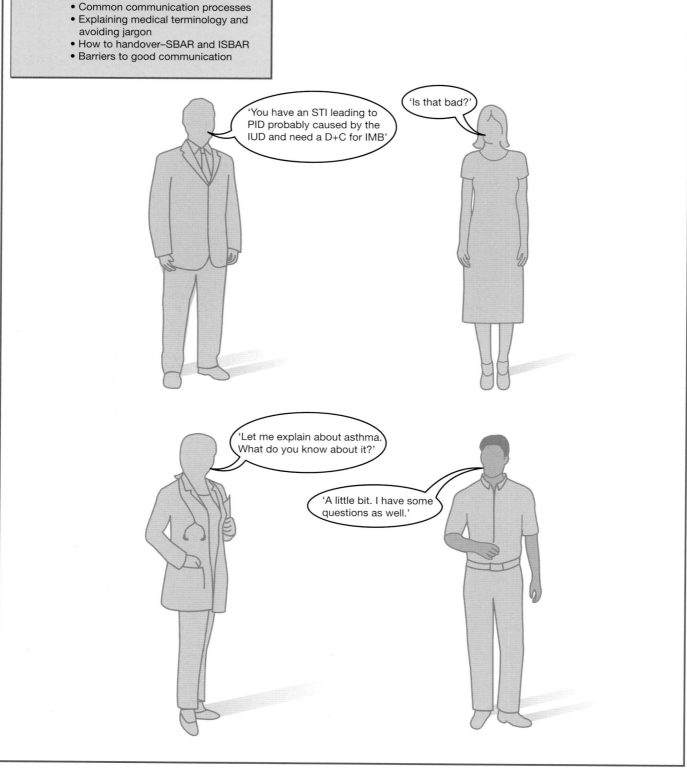

# Oral communication

This chapter focuses on oral communication: face-to-face, telephone and increasingly via multi-media.

## Why communication is important?

Research shows that good communication leads to more accurate diagnosis, greater patient satisfaction, increased rates of patient adherence to medication regimes, a reduction in stress and anxiety and enhanced doctors' well-being (Silverman et al., 2005).

---

Dr. Peter Nguyen is a doctor in training in a busy city hospital currently working on an acute medical ward. On a typical day he communicates with several new patients on admission; several patients he has been looking after for a few days, two of whom he speaks to before discharge to home; three family members; two senior doctors and two junior doctors including for hand over at the end of his shift; one general practitioner on the phone; nurses; a hospital pharmacist; staff in the biochemistry, haematology and microbiology laboratories; a radiographer and a physiotherapist.

---

Communication skills are an important component of medical training but tend to concentrate on patient–professional interactions in the early years. Yet communication, as Dr. Nguyen's example above shows, is multi-faceted and involves many different people for many different purposes. Some of these purposes are

- Eliciting a patient's history
- Explaining what happens during particular investigations such as gastroscopy, an MRI, etc.
- Discussing the meaning of test results
- Discussing management options
- Answering questions about medication
- Presenting a patient history to a senior colleague
- Speaking to a GP about a mutual patient's condition
- Explaining a patient's condition to her family
- Breaking bad news
- Obtaining informed consent
- Discussing a patient's condition with another health professional
- Comforting a distressed patient
- Disclosing an error to a senior colleague
- Working with an interpreter

All of the above, while different in content, have similar processes to consider. Consider which are appropriately or inappropriately carried out face-to-face, via telephone or multi-media.

## Common communication processes

Communication is a two-way process and involves **active listening** as well as talking. You will learn a lot about, and have time to practise, active listening in communication skills sessions. Being professional involves introducing yourself, showing respect and checking understanding after giving information. Medical students tend to pick up medical and professional jargon early in their training and need to be mindful that they have to adapt their language depending on the situation. Such jargon, including acronyms, is professional

---

Think and practise explaining the following to patients as well as considering what other words you could/might use in diverse circumstances and why:
- MI (myocardial infarction)
- ESR (erythrocyte sedimentation rate)
- Hepatitis B
- DRE (digital rectal examination)
- Haemorrhoids
- PSA (prostate-specific antigen)
- What aspirin does

---

shorthand and may add to the mystique surrounding medicine. However students and professionals also need to be careful of appearing patronising and 'talking down' to people. Patients and their families will vary in the extent of their health literacy – their ability to understand and make use of information about their health and treatment options. It is very important to check understanding frequently – this applies to all interaction within health care.

## Handover – SBAR and ISBAR

Doctors cannot be available 24 hours a day – they have to hand over patients at the end of a shift or to another specialist team. SBAR is an acronym and mnemonic to enhance patient safety in the handover process. It stands for Situation, Background, Assessment and Recommendation. Some institutions use ISBAR, where I is 'identify'.

---

Dr. Moira Dent is handing over a patient from the emergency department to Dr. Nguyen. She says
'This is Moira Dent, ED resident. I am admitting Deepak Patel a 73-year-old man, d.o.b. 12.6.1940, with a 2-day history of worsening shortness of breath, fever and purulent sputum. He has COPD and type 2 diabetes. His CXR shows a left-sided pneumonia. He requires IV antibiotics and blood glucose monitoring'.

---

How does this match the ISBAR process? Is there any other information that Dr. Nguyen requires?

## Barriers to good communication

There are many reasons for poor and miscommunication. The following are just a few:
- Lack of training for diverse situations
- Workload pressures
- Lack of time
- Communication not being seen as a priority
- Lack of a common language
- Lack of respect for colleagues
- Tiredness
- Stress
- Physical barriers such as deafness or dysphasia
- Noisy environment
- Being target driven

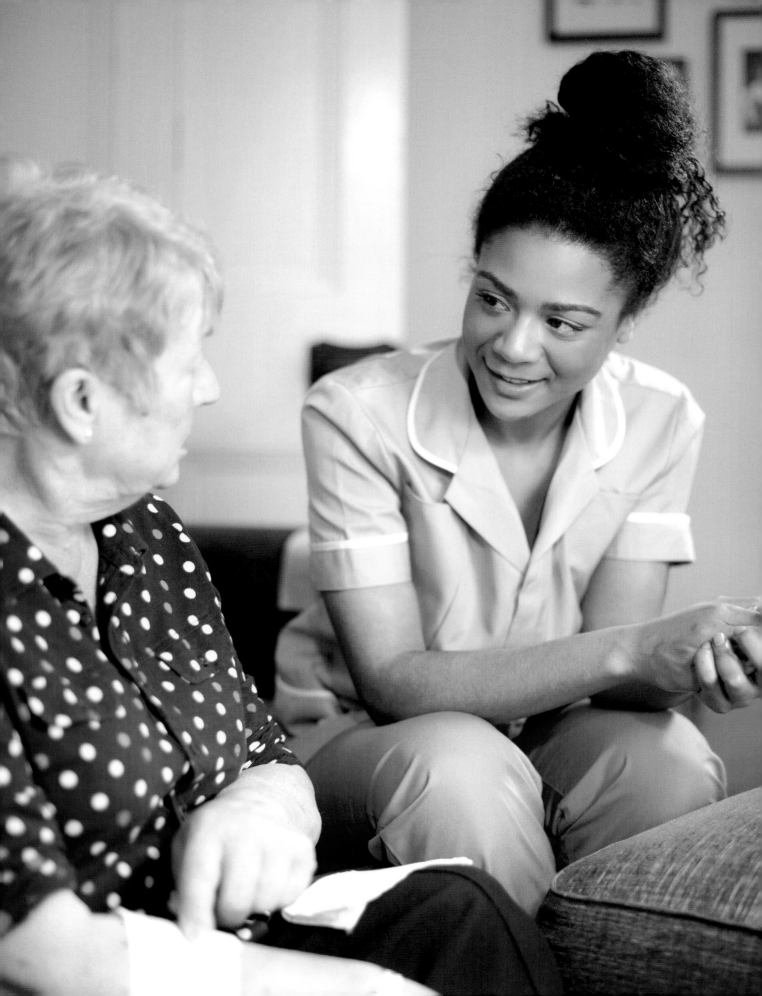

# Working with others

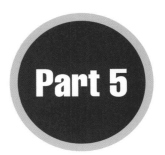

**Part 5**

## Chapters

# 33 Written communication

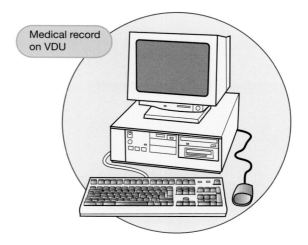

Medical record on VDU

## Be careful what you sign

Dr Gillespie is a junior doctor in a general practice. He has been treating Jack Smith for a broken finger sustained in a fight. The fracture is now healed. Jack asks the doctor to sign a medical certificate to say he is not fit to work for another week; he says the finger is still painful. He has been offered the chance of a beach holiday and thinks it will aid his recuperation. What is the professional course of action for Dr Gillespie?

## A referral letter from a doctor to a physiotherapist:

Dear Michael
Thank you for seeing 15 year-old Michael with his bad knees. Please manage as you think appropriately.
Ken.

**What information should be included in a referral letter?**

# Written communication and care

This chapter focuses on written communication in relation to patient care. Much of what is written now is stored, processed and transmitted electronically. Handwritten documents are less common and have problems relating to legibility and permanency.

## Why written communication is important?

Committing information to paper or on an electronic device should be viewed as making a permanent record of that information. In relation to patient details, writing forms part of the historical record and should not be altered at a later date unless the alterations are obvious and the reasons for change noted, such as a problem with accuracy.

As not all professional–professional and patient–professional interactions can be face to face, health care delivery relies on written communication for

- The medical record which will be seen by many people
- Hospital discharge and out-patient letters
- Referrals between professionals
- Test results
- Medical certificates and reports
- Passage of information both ways between patient and professional – for example, advice for patients on self-care following discharge from hospital
- Requests for information from third parties such as insurance companies or employers

These interactions may occur via surface post ('snail mail'), email or hand delivery, or as part of an electronic record system.

Health care documents are part of the legal record. They may be used in complaints/court cases/disciplinary proceedings. You may rely on them to prove your actions. It is important to remember that if you do not record what you have done, as soon as you have done it, there is no audit trail and it may be difficult to prove what you think you did in the future.

## Medical records – patient notes

> Dr. Valerie da Costa is a junior doctor in a busy city hospital currently working on a paediatric ward. She admitted 10-year-old Mohamed Hakim with fever and headache five hours ago. Mohamed is now fitting and looks extremely unwell. He has a rash suggestive of meningococcal septicaemia on his thighs. His parents say that the rash was present before he came in but that they were not asked about this. The paediatric registrar asks Valerie if she had checked for a rash on admission. She says that she did but she has not written in the notes 'no rash seen' and has not recorded asking the patients about a rash. The registrar stresses that it is vital to document important negative signs and symptoms as the parents have a good case to suggest that the diagnosis was not considered and was missed on admission.

While patient handover may be done orally there is not time to cover a patient's full medical history in this way. The medical record, which in some instances may go back many years, is of major importance for team-based care and when care is passed from one team to another. Most records are now computer-based (the EHR or electronic health record), while patient held records (the EPR or electronic patient record) and patient portals (cloud-based access to records) are becoming more common. It is impossible for most people to remember every detail about their prior illnesses, dates of screening tests, blood results, vaccination history, etc. Many patients cannot list their medication accurately ('I am on the little yellow pills nurse') or are unclear about diagnoses. (Some of these problems relate of course to poor communication from professionals in the past.)

Legally patients have access to their records in most circumstances even if they do not hold them personally, and therefore, it is important to remember not to write disparaging comments about patients in their notes – this is very unprofessional. Many health professionals choose to share notes informally without the patient having to make an official request for access. In clinics they may place the computer screen in such a way that the patient can see it. Some doctors dictate or write referral letters while the patient is present – this allows the patient to correct any misinformation and to know what the person to whom they are being referred has been told.

Sharing information about patients for the purpose of providing care is important and does not need formal consent from the patient, but it is courteous to remind patients that 'I will be writing to your GP to inform them of your admission and management plan'. However, the confidential health record should only be accessed by people directly involved in that patient's care. Written consent is required to share information with outside agencies such as insurance companies.

## Electronic communication

Email and text messaging are increasingly being used as a means of communication within health care; e.g. patients being reminded about appointment via text (SMS). Patients and professionals need to share a clear understanding of what information can be shared in this way, accessibility and response times. Emails tend to be more informal than typed letters – always remember to read through them carefully, check the recipient and pause before pressing send. Do not send anything in an email you would not want another person to see.

## Health informatics

Health informatics is concerned with the acquisition, storage, retrieval and communication of information in health care. It encompasses written communication and research into the methods of information transfer between all parties involved in patient care and the institutions in which they are involved. This is a growing branch of health care, as e-health and telemedicine become more prevalent, adding complexity to interactions while hopefully improving the actual communication processes.

# 34 Teamwork and interprofessional collaborative practice

- Definitions of teamwork and collaborative practice
- What helps teams function well
- How teams form

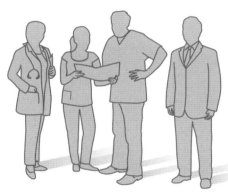

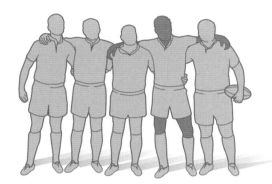

John, Julie, Mohammed, Aisha, Sarah and Kelly are second year students in a problem-based learning (PBL) course. They have not worked together before as there are new PBL groups each year. They also have an unfamiliar facilitator who is very hands-off and encourages them to work through problems with minimal input from herself. Three of the group struggle as they have been used to facilitators in the previous year who have been very directive. The other three are very comfortable with the way of working. The group struggles to work together; Julie and Sarah in particular become very critical of their colleagues' lack of preparation

- Whose responsibility is it to ensure the group begins to work well together?
- When does a group become a team?
- What would you do in this situation to ensure the group functions well?
- What lessons can you learn from this experience that have relevance for health care practice?

'Interprofessional collaboration is the process of developing and maintaining effective interprofessional working relationships with learners, practitioners, patients/clinics/families and communitities to enable optimal health outcomes. Elements of collaboration include respect, trust, shared decision making, and partnerships.'
Canadian Interprofessional Health Collaborative (CIHC)

Marie is a junior doctor working in mental health. She is talking to Don, a 56-year old man with depression in the day hospital. Don also has high blood pressure and is overweight. He tells Marie that in the last fortnight he has had interactions with the consultant psychiatrist, a community psychiatric nurse, a dietician and his general practitioner

# The importance of teamwork

Health care delivery in the 21st century in economically developed countries is multi-faceted, complex, often highly specialised and frequently carried out by teams of people – from varying disciplines and health professions. Patients with long-term conditions, such as cardiovascular disease, diabetes, dementia, cancer and mental health problems, interact with a large number of different health and social care professionals. Patients may be referred across locations (from primary to secondary care) and disciplines (from cardiology to radiology and surgery for example). They will also consult with doctors, nurses, pharmacists and allied health professionals. Some of these professionals will work in obvious co-located teams and some will work in looser collaborations.

# Definitions

> A team is a small number of people with complementary skills, who are committed to a common purpose, performance, goals and approach, for which they are mutually accountable.
>
> High performance team members are...committed to one another. Hammick et al. (2009, p. 39)
>
> Collaborative practice happens when multiple health workers from different professional backgrounds work together with patients, families, carers and communities to deliver the highest quality of care. It allows health workers to engage any individual whose skills can help achieve local health goals. Canadian Interprofessional Health Collaborative (2010)

## Your experience of teamwork

Think about your own experience of teamwork and being a member of a team – this may include a sports team, a choir or orchestra, a problem-based learning group, etc.

• What distinguishes a well-functioning team from one that is dysfunctional?
• What skills do team members need to enable a team to work well?
• What similarities and differences are there likely to be between the teams you have been a member of and a health care team?
• What do you need to develop to be able to work in a health care team?

## Characteristics of functioning teams

Three conditions have been defined as necessary for functioning teamwork (Dawson et al., 2007):

> 1. Clear objectives that are known to all members.
> 2. Team members work closely together to achieve these objectives.
> 3. There are regular meetings to review team effectiveness and discuss how it can be improved.

In addition, there needs to be a shared commitment between team members and clarity about each other's roles and responsibilities. Team members should agree their processes for working together and discuss each other's values. As you will appreciate from your own experience of teamwork, all members need to actively participate in discussions and tasks, and regular debriefing to evaluate team performance is important. Members should respect one another and deal with conflict as it arises. We can sum this up by saying that team members should behave professionally to one another and professionally as a team.

# Working in a 'new' team

As a student you are likely to work in teams that are newly formed – you may not know or have worked with other team members before. One description of the stages new teams may go through is shown in the box below. Does this fit with your experience?

> **Stages of team development (from Tuckman and Jensen, 1977)**
> • **Forming** – members are polite as they get to know each other; this is the stage of sounding each other out. Here the team should define group rules and discuss values and goals.
> • **Storming** – members may question the defined goals and values as they get to know each other better and be more relaxed. Some members may reveal attitudes that do not resonate with the team's defined values. There may be tension and outright conflict, particularly if some members are not participating fully in team tasks.
> • **Norming** – respect develops and communication is enhanced as team members develop better understanding of each other.
> • **Performing** – there is effective and productive work; the team begins to meet its goals.

# Joining a ready-formed team

In the clinical environment you are more likely to become a member of an already formed and functioning team. How will you ensure that you fit in with your team members? As a junior professional you are likely to need time to understand the dynamics of the team and the roles of the people within it. You are also likely to be a member of more than one team – and will collaborate with many different people while providing patient care. Certainly in your career you will encounter poorly performing teams which have the characteristics show below:

## Characteristics of dysfunctioning teams

> • Absence of trust
> • Fear of conflict
> • Lack of commitment
> • Avoidance of accountability
> • Inattention to results (Lencioni, 2002)

See Chapter 24 for the concept of in-groups and its relevance to teams.

# 35 Leadership and followership

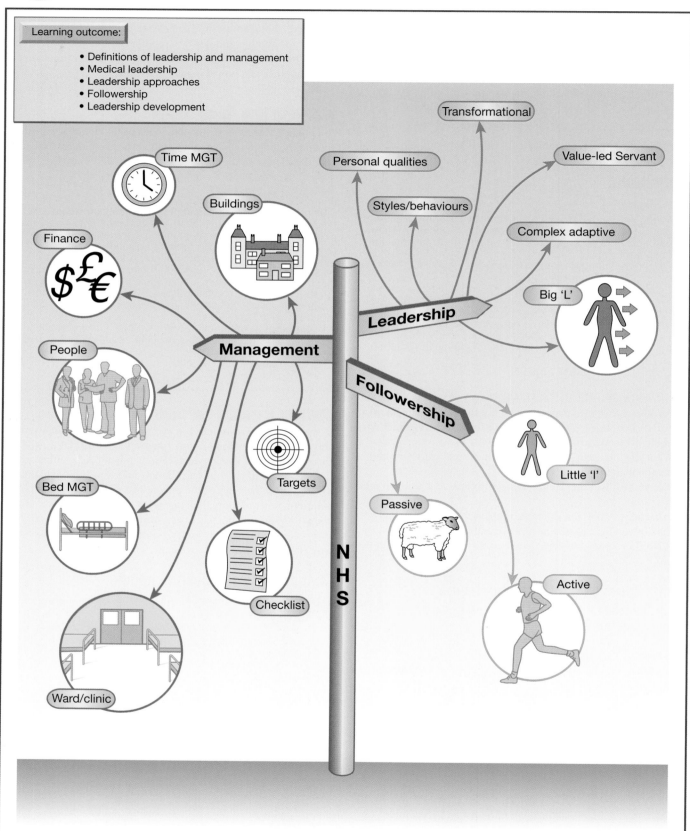

## Definition

Leadership can be defined as 'a process whereby an individual influences a group of individuals to achieve a common goal' (Northouse, 2010, p. 3).

## Leadership and management

Health care management has been described as 'the dark side' (Spurgeon et al., 2011) and until relatively recently many clinicians have been unwilling to take on management positions. However, management and leadership are both vital to ensuing that things happen as planned, as well as providing impetus for change and direction. Management is about planning, providing stability and order (doing things right), whereas leadership is about change, setting direction and adaptability (doing the right thing). Organisations, teams or situations need both leadership and management in varying amounts depending on the context.

## What is leadership about?

On a day-to-day basis, clinical leadership involves working with patients and families, medical colleagues, managers, other health professionals and learners to achieve good outcomes for patients. Leadership involves decision-making, team leadership, self-management and high-level communication skills and is therefore closely aligned with other professional attributes and behaviours (see Chapter 15). Leadership skills, models and theories (and your own development) can be thought of in terms of three overlapping categories (Swanwick and McKimm, 2014):

- *Intrapersonal* – focussing on the personal qualities or personality of the leader – involves getting to know yourself and developing self-insight, understanding your strengths and weaknesses and how you respond under pressure;
- *Interpersonal* – relating to the interaction of the leader with others – working in teams, with other health workers, patients and families, how do others see you?;
- *Organisational/system-wide* – leadership in relation to the organisation or system – involves learning about and understanding the wider health system, your organisation, politics and processes and how change and improvement may be managed.

## Leadership approaches

The main approaches to understanding leadership are as follows:
- Trait theories – focussing on personality traits and a list of 'qualities' (e.g. integrity, charisma, approachability, concern);
- Style theories – how the leader behaves in different situations (e.g. authoritative, consultative), takes account that leadership can be modified and learned;
- Transactional and transformational – transactional relates to management and involves exchange of effort for reward (e.g. you work for the NHS and you get paid). Transformational leadership is about leaders inspiring and motivating others towards higher order goals or values. Whilst this is appealing in health care, the realities of a managed system with targets and performance measures can lead to cynicism;

- Collaborative, shared, distributed and collective leadership – these approaches look at leadership 'at all levels' of an organisation and consider that it is only by working together that real change and improvement will be made;
- Adaptive leadership – is about working in complex, uncertain times and adapting ways of working to develop solutions to new or 'wicked' problems;
- Eco-leadership, value-led, servant and moral leadership – all involve 'making a difference' through engaging with the moral purpose and values of organisations, and looking to environmental and societal sustainability.

## Followership

Leaders need to have people who 'follow' them and the concept of followership can be helpful, particularly for learners. Kelley (1988) distinguishes between four groups:
- *Passive followers* – he calls these 'sheep', they do as they are told;
- *Active followers* – questioning and supportive;
- *Little 'l' leaders* – leading in small ways, leadership at all levels;
- *Big 'L' leaders* – senior leaders, leading major situations, projects or organisations.

---

- You are on a busy acute surgical ward and have a list of things to do and patients to see.
- What management skills do you use to ensure you get everything done properly?
- If an emergency occurs, you might need leadership or followership skills? What skills will you need to use?

---

The concepts of little 'l' leaders or 'project champions' can help students or doctors in training who are engaging in service improvement projects to see where they 'fit' in the project or system (Bohmer, 2010). Becoming an 'expert' in your project or initiative helps build credibility when power and influence is relatively low because of position in the organisation and medical hierarchy (Till et al., 2014).

## Leadership development

Since 2008, increased attention has been paid to medical leadership and now many opportunities exist for students, doctors in training and practising doctors to 'learn leadership'.

The NHS Healthcare Leadership Model (www.leadershipacademy.nhs.uk/discover/leadershipmodel) provides a competency and development framework for all health workers. Students' leadership roles might include leading a society or event or taking part in a service improvement project or audit. Many undergraduate curricula include some elements of leadership and all doctors in training are now required to undertake leadership workshops or e-learning courses. If you are very interested in leadership, some academic programmes in clinical leadership are available including opportunities for becoming a 'leadership fellow' and undertaking postgraduate qualifications. The Faculty of Medical Leadership and Management (FMLM) welcomes students and doctors in training (as well as other professionals) and provides many opportunities for learning and presenting on leadership and access to a wide range of resources.

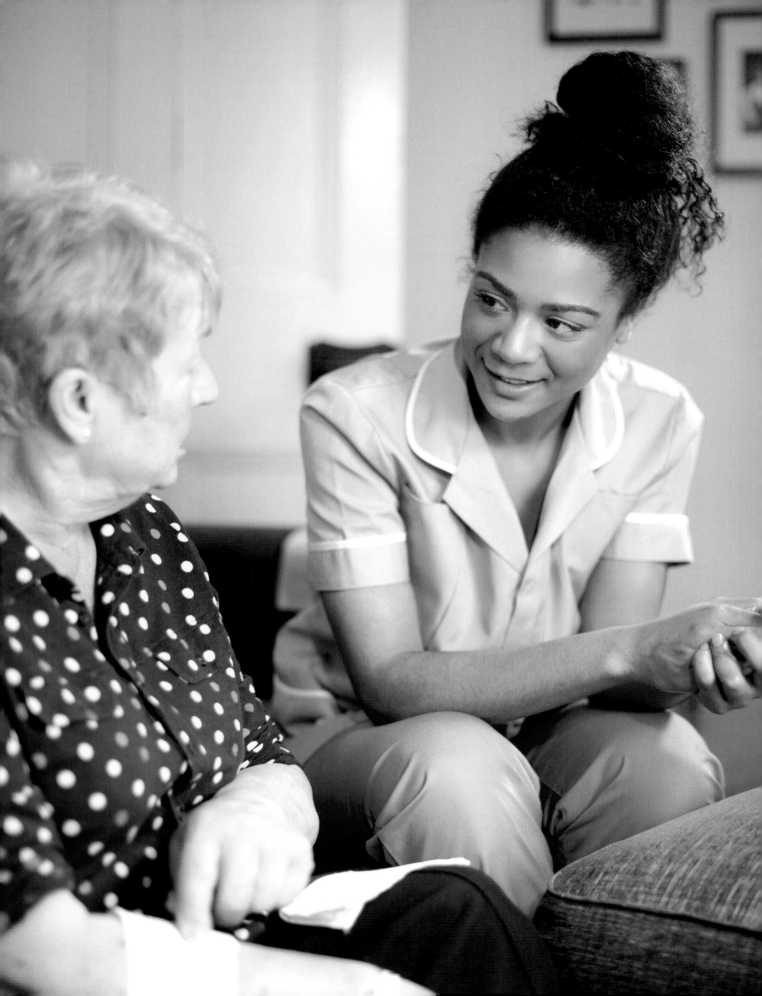

# Professional issues and dilemmas

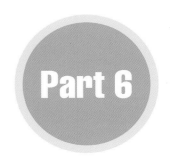

**Part 6**

## Chapters

# 36 When things go wrong

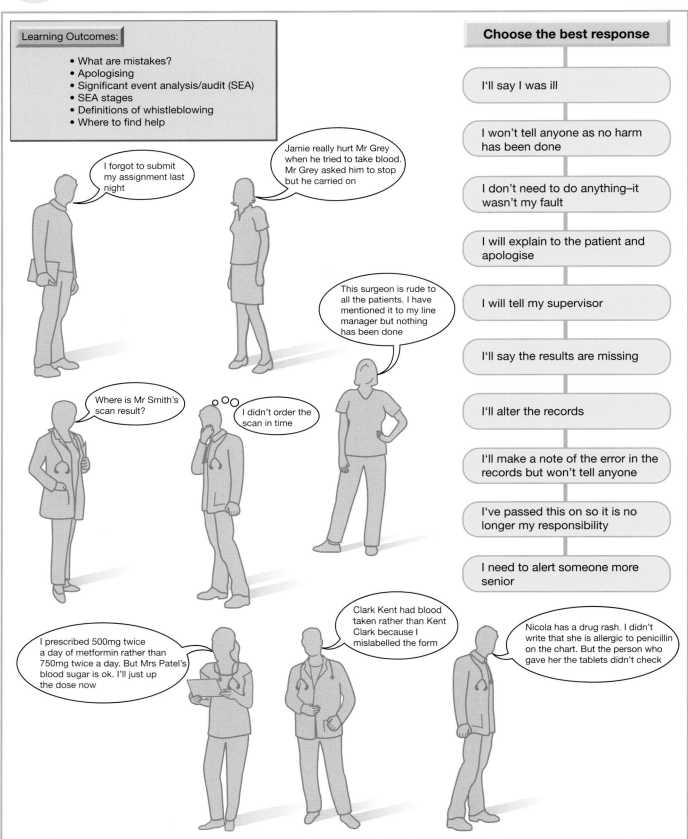

**Learning Outcomes:**

- What are mistakes?
- Apologising
- Significant event analysis/audit (SEA)
- SEA stages
- Definitions of whistleblowing
- Where to find help

n Chapter 37 we discuss the process for making and dealing with formal complaints against health professionals and students. In this chapter we look at other ways in which unprofessional behaviour may be detected and ways of responding to this, when either an official complaint is not considered necessary or appropriate, or the official system fails to act in some way.

## Making mistakes

Everyone makes mistakes because we are all human beings and can't know or be able to do everything. Mistakes are usually incidents that we come to regret and are unplanned, whereas actions that we know are wrong and yet still carry out are malicious in intent. In health care, of course, mistakes may have devastating effects (see chapter 26 on patient safety) but frequently they have only local or personal consequences. If a mistake goes undetected or can be rectified without anyone knowing, is there a professional duty to report it? Covering up a mistake or leaving someone else to take the blame is certainly unprofessional and morally suspect in any situation. Generally the fault is then the cover up rather than the mistake itself.

As mistakes are common we need to learn from them: why did this occur; how might I prevent it in future; what do I need to learn to ensure this does not happen again? We should also be careful that fear of making mistakes does not impair our performance.

> Think of a situation in which you have made a mistake. Who did you tell and why? How did you feel? What did you do/need to do to try to set things right? What did you learn from the experience? How did/might your experience and learning help you in the future in a professional context?

In professional development sessions you may discuss mistakes and how you should deal with your own personal examples. A role play or simulated patient scenario could involve you apologising to a colleague or a patient following a mistake. However difficult an apology is, it is far better than concealment and living with your actions preying on your mind. Patients are far less likely to make formal complaints if they receive sincere apologies that help them understand what has gone wrong.

In clinical situations mistakes should be reported to your supervisor, in an emergency you need to contact the most appropriate person to help rectify the resulting problems. Do not try to deal with things on your own – your emotional state is likely to make things worse and cloud your judgement. If you see someone else make a mistake you should encourage them to report the incident, but advise them that you have a duty to do this if they do not.

> What sorts of mistakes need reporting? Have you ever seen incidents that you felt uncomfortable about? Do you know within your institution who you should report mistakes to?

## Significant event analysis/audit

A significant event is one thought by anyone in the clinical team or wider location to be significant in relation to the care of patients or the conduct of the organization (Pringle et al., 1995). The significant event analysis/audit (SEA) should involve all relevant parties learning from each other and contributing to the discussion. In practice an SEA has seven stages:

> **Stage 1**: A staff member becomes aware of a significant event and makes it a priority for a meeting and discussion.
> **Stage 2**: Before and during the meeting, information is collected and collated from all involved.
> **Stage 3**: Facilitated meeting – discussion should be open, honest and non-threatening. The aim is not to apportion blame but to explore what has happened and to learn from this, in order to prevent an occurrence in the future.
> **Stage 4**: Analysis of the event: what happened; why did circumstances unfold as they did; what may be learnt from the events and what, if anything, needs to be changed.
> **Stage 5**: Agree an action plan and answer to the question 'What is the chance of this event happening again?'
> **Stage 6**: Minutes written up and circulated in confidence to appropriate personnel.
> **Stage 7**: Report, share and review (see NHS, 2008).

## Whistleblowing

Whistleblowing is the disclosure by a person, usually an employee, to the public or to the authorities, of negligence, cover-ups, mismanagement, corruption, illegality, bullying and malpractice at their workplace. It is also referred to as 'disclosure in the public interest' (www.gov.uk/whistleblowing/overview). Organisations may have a whistleblowing policy: this should be checked with HR (human resources). A whistleblower should try to refer the matter to their employer first but if there are compelling reasons not to do so, they should contact a prescribed person. Reasons to go outside the workplace include concern that the employer will cover up the problem; fear of subsequent unfair treatment or dismissal; not acting after initial reporting. Lists of prescribed persons/bodies in health care are available but are frequently updated so need checking before action.

In the United Kingdom, there is a helpline for NHS and social care staff: www.wbhelpline.org.uk/. In Australia there is an association for whistleblowers: www.whistleblowers.org.au/

However, many people are still wary of speaking out because of high-profile cases in which whistleblowers have been treated badly for their actions and labelled them 'career suicide' (Guardian Professional, 2013).

> Are you aware of any whistleblowing incidents in your health service? What are the common themes and what is the response? You may wish to Google the following: the Francis report of the Mid-Staffordshire public inquiry; the Kennedy report of the Bristol Royal Infirmary; investigations into Camden and Campbelltown hospitals (New South Wales), Canberra Hospital and King Edward Memorial Hospital (Western Australia); the Patel affair at the Bundaberg hospital (Queensland).

# 37 Dealing with complaints

**Learning outcome:**

- Why people complain
- The complaints process
- Complaints against medical students
- Fitness to practise hearings

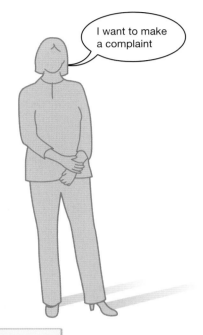

A 2010 USA study found that 27.4% of final year medical students surveyed had engaged in cheating or dishonest behaviour (Dyrbye et al. 2010)

Why do some unprofessional behaviours become more acceptable?

*Health Care Professionalism at a Glance*, First Edition. Jill Thistlethwaite and Judy McKimm.
© 2016 by John Wiley & Sons, Ltd. Published 2016 by John Wiley & Sons, Ltd.

## Reasons for complaints

Have you ever felt like complaining for services you have received? Such services may include at a restaurant (poor food and rude waiters); in a shop (overcharged); for a commodity (slower downloads on the Internet than advertised; product breaks after one use). These events happen frequently in our lives but there is a tipping point at which we feel 'enough is enough' and decide to take action. What do you think triggers patients to complain about health professionals and the care they receive?

By far the main reason patients make complaints about their doctors and other health professionals is related to treatments and investigations, but poor communication and lack of respect are also frequent problems. We know ourselves that we are less likely to lodge a complaint when something goes wrong in any situation if we are listened to, a full explanation is given, an apology is made and, if necessary, compensation is offered. Patients and families on the whole expect honesty and integrity from their health care professionals. Frequently they make a complaint in order to know what exactly went wrong and why.

### Some statistics

In the United Kingdom, complaints about doctors received by the GMC have been on the rise since 2007, with an increase of 24% since 2011, and 100% in the last 6 years (GMC, 2013e). Most complaints come from the public, with a smaller number from employers (e.g. hospitals) and other doctors. The GMC, however, stresses that the number of complaints is low compared to the number of registered doctors and that globally there is a trend towards more service users making complaints against all health professionals not just doctors. This increase may be due to a combination of changing attitudes to professionals (which some commentators believe is a sign of health care becoming another consumer commodity) and improved systems for identifying problems and the complaints process.

## The complaints process

Patients are advised to complain to the place and the professionals where they received care. Often people want explanations or an apology and this may be sorted out to their satisfaction at a local level: at their general practice (through the practice manager), the hospital (public or private) or at a clinic. For more serious concerns about doctors, such that the patient or family wonder if a doctor is fit to practise, the complaint should be made to the GMC (or national registration board of the country, such as AHPRA in Australia; the relevant state's medical society or licensing board in the United States; the local provincial/territorial Ministry of Health in Canada).

The GMC initially triages the complaint and decides whether action is required. This may be by advising that the matter is dealt with locally by referring to the doctor's employer or practice; issuing a warning to the doctor; stipulating that the doctor requires more training or supervision; referral to a fitness to practise panel which may decide to suspend or remove the doctor's registration.

The GMC does not fine a doctor or help with claims for compensation. If a patient or family wishes to receive payment for mistakes or poor treatment, they have to seek legal advice.

Note also that **all doctors** must act when they believe that a colleague is giving cause for concern in relation to patient safety, or if a patient's care or dignity is at risk. This is a professional duty.

---

**Referral to the GMC complaints procedure if a doctor**
- Makes serious or frequent mistakes in relation to diagnoses, carrying out procedures (e.g. surgery), or prescribing
- Fails or refuses to examine a patient
- Commits fraud or is dishonest
- Breaches a patient's confidentiality
- Commits a serious criminal offence (doctor should be reported to the police as well)
- (GMC, 2012b).

---

## Complaints about medical students

Are you aware of the system within your medical school for the reporting of unprofessional behaviour by a medical student? You should have been advised of this during orientation.

## Fitness to practise

The GMC states that 'medical students have certain privileges and responsibilities different from those of other students. Because of this, different standards of professional behaviour are expected of them' (GMC, 2009a, p. 4). This book describes and discusses this professional behaviour. Fitness to practise decisions are made locally within the medical school or university once concerns have been raised by tutors, clinicians, peers, patients or the community. The questions a fitness to practise panel considers are (GMC, 2009a):
- Has a student's behaviour harmed patients or put patients at risk of harm?
- Has a student shown a deliberate or reckless disregard of professional and clinical responsibilities towards patients or colleagues?
- Is a student's health or impairment compromising patient safety?
- Has a student abused a patient's trust or violated a patient's autonomy or other fundamental rights?
- Has a student behaved dishonestly, fraudulently, or in a way designed to mislead or harm others?

---

The fitness to practise panel at Anytown Medical School is considering the cases of third-year student BD and final year student FH. BD was seen using his mobile phone to take pictures of the end of semester MCQ examination. FH has been reported by a patient's wife for being rude to her husband during a physical examination. The patient, whose BMI was 34, was complaining of chest, back and knee pain. The student allegedly said 'what do you expect when you are obese'.

Do you feel these cases are comparable? Some of BD's fellow students remarked: but nearly everyone does that!

---

## 38 Case studies: professional dilemmas

All health professional students and qualified professionals come across professional issues or dilemmas regularly. Sometimes these directly involve you, at other times you may observe actions (or inactions) that you feel uncomfortable about. A lot of these situations come about when we feel we should speak out or say something but we feel we can't because of power imbalances, fear of being seen as 'difficult' or because patients and families are around. Below are a series of different scenarios representing professional issues. For each of the following scenarios think about or discuss the professionalism issues involved and what you should (or could) do to deal with them.

### Case 1

A clinical tutor draws you aside after a bedside teaching session. She says she was in a local bar over the weekend having a quiet drink and became aware of a group of young men who appeared to be drinking heavily. They became louder and louder as the evening went on. A few of them began to use lewd language towards three women at the next table. Eventually they were asked to leave the bar by one of the bar staff. As the men left, the clinical tutor recognized at least two as medical students – one of whom she identifies as you. She asks you to explain yourself and says she is thinking about reporting you for a breach of professionalism. She also asks you the name of the other student. How would you respond? Is professional behaviour only required when you are 'at work'?

### Case 2

Joshua Radcliffe is a third-year medical student who is spending a morning with an anaesthetist, Dr. Rudd. Joshua has spent some time in the clinical skills laboratory and has been deemed competent at inserting venous cannula into dummy arms over the past few weeks. He informs the anaesthetist that he hopes to cannulate a 'real' patient. Dr. Rudd asks the next patient if she is happy for a medical student to insert her venous line. She consents but Joshua wonders if he should inform her that this would be his first time with a 'real' arm. Perhaps she wouldn't be so happy with that.

### Case 3

You are a first-year medical student with a congenital heart problem, which you have declared to the medical school administration but few other people are aware of this. You see a cardiologist twice a year for a check-up. During a clinical skills session the same cardiologist is a guest clinician and he is talking about the cardiovascular system examination. He plays audio recordings of various heart murmurs. He then suggests that the group could listen to your heart as an example of a 'good mitral murmur'.

### Case 4

You are a member of a group of six second-year students from different professions who are carrying out a community-based project. The assessment for this task is a group presentation for which an overall mark will be awarded to the group. One of your group members, though present at every meeting, has not really been engaged in the process and has had little input into the presentation. The remaining five of you are unhappy that this member will receive the same marks as the rest of you.

Should an exercise of this kind be self, peer and facilitator marked for each student separately? What are the advantages and disadvantages of self and peer assessment?

### Case 5

Rosa Sanchez is concerned about her medical school friend Huan Wang. They were both attached to a general practice for 4 weeks 2 months ago in a rural area. During that time Huan was asked to see a 25-year-old farmer with eczema and then discuss the case with the GP. The man asked Huan out to dinner a day after the consultation and the pair of them spent a lot of time together during the rest of the rotation. The farmer has now appeared in town and wants to continue the relationship.

### Case 6

Morris McAllister is a first-year doctor working in the Emergency Department of a busy hospital. While preparing an ampoule to give an injection to a patient he cuts his index finger, which begins to bleed. He quickly puts a plaster on it and carries on. Later he is percussing a child's chest. The mother points out that his finger is bleeding and that the blood is smearing onto her child's back.

### Case 7

You are a registered nurse on a general medical ward. There are always a lot of different health professional students passing through, talking to and examining patients, having teaching, etc. One particular female student has been concerning you. She seems to hang behind the others, with no confidence and you have never seen her approach a patient by herself. You take her aside one day and ask if anything is wrong. She bursts into tears and says she doesn't like sick people and is scared she will make them more ill. She admits she is not sleeping or eating well.

*Health Care Professionalism at a Glance*, First Edition. Jill Thistlethwaite and Judy McKimm.
© 2016 by John Wiley & Sons, Ltd. Published 2016 by John Wiley & Sons, Ltd.

# References

Alaszewski A (1995) Restructuring health and welfare professions in the United Kingdom. In: T Johnson, G Larkin, M Saks (eds.), *Health Professions and the State in Europe*. London: Routledge, pp. 55–74.

Al-Eraky MM, Donkers J, Wajid G, van Merrienboer JJG (2014) A Delphi study of medical professionalism in Arabian countries: the Four-Gates model. *Med Teach*, 36, S8–S16.

Allport GW (1979) *The Nature of Prejudice*, 25th anniversary edition. Reading, MA: Addison-Wesley Publishing Company.

Arnold R (2005) *Empathic Intelligence: Teaching, Learning, Relating.* Sydney: UNSW Press.

Becher T, Trowler P (2001) *Academic Tribes and Territories: Intellectual Enquiry and the Culture of Disciplines,* 2nd edition. Buckingham: SHRE and Open University Press.

Becker HS, Geer B, Hughes EC, Strauss AL (1961) *Boys in White: Student Culture in Medical School.* Transaction Publishers.

Benner P (1984) *From Novice to Expert: Excellence and Power in Clinical Nursing.* Menlo Park, CA: Addison-Wesley.

Bohmer R (2010) Leadership with a small 'l'. *Br Med J*, 340, c483.

Borton T (1970) *Reach, Teach and Touch.* London: McGraw Hill.

Boud D, Keogh R, Walker D (1989) *Reflection: Turning Experience into Learning.* London: Kogan Page.

Boulet J, van Zanten M (2014) Ensuring high quality patient care: the role of accreditation, licensure, specialty certification and revalidation in medicine. *Med Educ*, 48, 75–86.

Brimstone R, Thistlethwaite JE, Quirk F (2007) Health help-seeking behaviour of medical students. *Med Educ*, 41, 74–83.

British Medical Association (BMA) (1998) *The Misuse of Alcohol and Other Drugs by Doctors. A Report of the Working Group on the Misuse of Alcohol and Other Drugs.* London: BMA.

Canadian Interprofessional Health Collaborative (2010) *A National Interprofessional Competency Framework*, http://www.cihc.ca/files/CIHC_IPCompetencies_Feb1210r.pdf

Chartered Society of Physiotherapy (2014) *What Is Professionalism?*, http://www.csp.org.uk/professional-union/professionalism/what-professionalism

Chen DC, Kirshenbaum DS, Kirshenbaum E, Aseltine RH (2012) Characterising changes in student empathy throughout medical school. *Med Teach*, 34, 305–311.

Clack GB, Allen J, Cooper D, Head JO (2004) Personality differences between doctors and their patients: implications for teaching of communication skills. *Med Educ*, 38, 177–186.

Clinical Governance Support Team (2007) *Guidance on the Role and Effective Use of Chaperones in Primary and Community Care Settings: Model Chaperone Framework*, http://www.lmc.org.uk/visageimages/guidance/2007/Chaperone_model%20framework.pdf

Coulter A, Entwistle V, Gilbert D (1999) Sharing decisions with patients: is the information good enough? *Br Med J*, 31, 318–322.

Crawley J (2005) *In at the Deep End – A Survival Guide for Teachers in Post Compulsory Education.* London: David Fulton.

Cruess RL, Cruess SR (2010) Professionalism is a generic term: practicing what we preach. *Med Teach*, 32(9), 713–714.

Cruess RR, Johnston S, Cruess RL (2004) Profession: a working definition for medical educators. *Teach Learn Med*, 16, 74–76.

Dawson JF, Yan X, West MA (2007) *Positive and Negative Effects of Team Working in Healthcare: Real and Pseudo-Teams and Their Impact on Safety.* Birmingham: Aston University.

Department of Health (DoH) (1991) *The Patient Charter.* London: DoH.

Dickinson D, Raynor DK (2003) Ask the patients – they may want to know more than you think. *Br Med J*, 327, 861.

Dubler NN (1992) Individual advocacy as a governing principle. *J Case Manag*, 13, 82–86.

Dyrbye LN, Massie FS Jr, Eacker A, Harper W, Power D, Durning SJ, Thomas MR, Moutier C, Satele D, Sloan J, Shanafelt TD (2010) Relationship between burnout and professional conduct and attitudes among US medical students. *J Am Med Assoc,* 304, 1173–1180.

Epstein RM (1999) Mindful practice. *J Am Med Assoc*, 282 (9): 833–839

Eraut M (2004) Informal learning in the workplace. *Stud Contin Educ*, 26 (2), 247–273.

Eva K, Macala C (2014) Multiple mini-interview test characteristics: 'tis better to ask candidates to recall than to imagine. *Med Educ*, 48(6), 604–613. doi:10.1111/medu.12402

Firth-Cozens J (2003) Doctors, their wellbeing and their stress. *Br Med J*, 326, 670–671.

Fulford KWM (2004) Ten principles of values-based practice. In: Radden J (ed.), *The Philosophy of Psychiatry: A Companion.* New York: Oxford University Press, pp. 205–234.

Galletly CA (2004) Crossing professional boundaries in medicine: the slippery slope to patient sexual exploitation. *Med J Aust*, 181, 380–383.

General Medical Council (GMC) (2009a) *Medical Students: Professional Values and Fitness to Practise.* London: GMC.

General Medical Council (GMC) (2009b) *Tomorrow's Doctors.* London: GMC.

General Medical Council (GMC) (2010) *Revalidation. A Statement of Intent.* London: GMC.

General Medical Council (GMC) (2012a) *How to Complain about a Doctor.* London: GMC.

General Medical Council (GMC) (2012b) *Raising and Acting on Concerns about Patient Safety.* London: GMC.

General Medical Council (GMC) (2012c) *Ready for Revalidation.* London: GMC.

General Medical Council (GMC) (2013a) *Financial and Commercial Arrangements and Conflicts of Interest.* London: GMC.

General Medical Council (GMC) (2013b) *Good Medical Practice.* London: GMC.

General Medical Council (GMC) (2013c) *Maintaining a Professional Boundary between You and Your Patient.* London: GMC.

General Medical Council (GMC) (2013d) *Supporting Students with Mental Health Conditions.* London: GMC.

General Medical Council (GMC) (2013e) *The State of Medical Education and Practice in the UK Report: 2013.* London: GMC.

Gibbs G (1988) *Learning by Doing: A Guide to Teaching and Learning Methods.* Oxford: Oxford Further Education Unit.

Guardian Professional (2013) *Duty of Candour: A Fear of Whistleblowing Still Pervades the NHS*, www.theguardian.com/healthcare-network/2013/dec/09/duty-candour-whistleblowing-pervades-nhs

Hafferty F (2004) Toward the operationalization of professionalism: a commentary. *Am J Bioeth*, 4 (2), 28–31.

Hafferty F, Franks R (1994) The hidden curriculum, ethics teaching and the structure of medical education. *Acad Med,* 69(11), 861–871.

Hammick M, Freeth D, Copperman J, Goodsman D (2009) *Being Interprofessional.* Cambridge: Polity Press.

Henning K, Ey S, Shaw D (1998) Perfectionism, the imposter phenomenon and psychological adjustment in medical, dental, nursing and pharmacy students. *Med Educ,* 23, 456–464.

Hilton SR, Slotnick HB (2005) Proto-professionalism: how professionalisation occurs across the continuum of medical education. *Med Educ,* 39, 58–65.

House RB (1948) Some college values are caught and not taught. *J Gen Educ,* 2 (3), 187–192.

Institute of Medicine (IOM) (1999) To Err is Human: Building a Safer Health System. The IOM Committee's first report. IOM.

Johnson TJ (1972) *Professions and Power.* London: Macmillan.

Jones R (2002) Declining altruism in medicine. *Br Med J,* 324, 625–625.

Joubert G, Steinberg H, Beylefeld A (2009) Guiding undergraduate medical students to use literature appropriately. *Med Educ,* 43, 1090.

Kelley RE (1988) In praise of followers. *Harv Bus Rev,* 66 (6), 142–148.

Kerridge I, Lowe M, McPhee J (2005) *Ethics and Law for the Health Professions,* 2nd edition. Sydney: The Federation Press.

Kessler D, Hamilton W (2004) Normalisation: horrible word, useful idea. *Br J Gen Pract,* 54, 163–164.

Khong E, Sim MG, Hulse G (2002) The identification and management of the drug impaired doctor. *Aust Fam Physician,* 31, 1097–1100.

Kleinman A, Benson P (2006) Anthropology in the clinic: the problem with cultural competency and how to fix it. *PLoS Med,* 3 (10), e294. doi:10.1371/journal.pmed.0030294

Lave J, Wenger E (1991) *Situated Learning: Legitimate Peripheral Participation.* Cambridge: University of Cambridge Press.

Lencioni P (2002) *The Five Dysfunctions of a Team.* Lafayette: The Table Group.

Livingstone DW (1999) Exploring the iceberg of adult learning: findings from the first Canadian survey of informal learning practices. *Can J Study Adult Educ,* 13 (2), 49–72.

Lown BA, Rosen J, Marttila J (2011) An agenda for improving compassionate care: a survey shows about half of patients say such care is missing. *Health Aff (Millwood),* 30 (9), 1772–1778.

Mayer J, Salovey P (1997) What is emotional intelligence? In P Salovey, DJ Sluyter (eds.), *Emotional Development and Emotional Intelligence: Educational Applications.* New York: Basic Books.

Mayer J, Salovey P, Caruso D, Sitarenios G (2003) Measuring emotional intelligence with the MSCEIT V2.0. *Emotion,* 3, 97–105.

McKimm J (2009) Assessing educational needs. *Multiprofessional Faculty Development.* NHS Health Education England. www.faculty.londondeanery.ac.uk/e-learning/assessing-educational-needs

McManus C, Dewberry C, Nicholson S, Dowell JS (2013) The UKCAT-12 study: educational attainment, aptitude test performance, demographic and socio-economic contextual factors as predictors of first year outcome in a cross-sectional collaborative study of 12 UK medical schools. *BMC Med,* 11, 244. doi:10.1186/1741-7015-11-244

Moon J (2004) *A Handbook of Reflective and Experiential Learning: Theory and Practice.* London: Routledge.

Morris, C, McKimm, J (2009) Becoming a digital tourist: a guide for clinical teachers. *The Clinical Teacher,* 6, 51-55.

National Patient Safety Foundation (NPSF) (2003) *The Role of the Patient Advocate: A Consumer Fact Sheet.* Boston, MA: NPSF. http://www.npsf.org

NHS (2008) www.nrls.npsa.nhs.uk/resources/?entryid45=61500>

NICE (National Institute for Health and Care Excellence) (2002) *Principles for Best Practice in Medical Audit.* Oxford: Radcliffe Medical Press.

Northouse PG (2010) *Leadership Theory and Practice.* London: Sage.

Nursing and Midwifery Board of Australia (2008) *Code of Professional Conduct for Nurses in Australia,* www.nursingmidwiferyboard.gov.au

Oriel K, Plane MB, Mundt M (2004) Family medicine residents and the imposter phenomenon. *Fam Med,* 36, 248–252.

Paice E, Heard S, Moss F (2002) How important are role models in making good doctors? *Br Med J,* 325, 707–710.

Patel P, Zed PJ (2002) Drug-related visits to the emergency department. How big is the problem? *Pharmacotherapy,* 22, 915–923.

Pringle M, Bradley CP, Carmichael C, Wallis H, Moore A (1995) *Significant Event Auditing.* Occasional Paper No.70. London: Royal College of General Practitioners.

Project of the ABIM Foundation, ACP-ASIM Foundation, and European Federation of Internal Medicine (2002) Medical professionalism in the new millennium: a physician charter. *Ann Intern Med,* 136, 243-246.

RCN Principles of Nursing Practice 2010b

Rees C, Monrouxe L, McDonald L (2013) Narrative, emotion and action: analysing 'most memorable' professionalism dilemmas. *Med Educ,* 47, 80–96.

RNAO (2007) *Professionalism in Nursing,* http://rnao.ca/bpg/guidelines/professionalism-nursing

Roberts LW, Warner TD, Carter D, Frank E, Ganzini L, Lyketsos C (2000) Caring for medical students as patients. *Acad Med,* 75, 272–277.

Roughead EE, Semple SJ (2009) Medication safety in acute care in Australia. *Aust New Zealand Health Policy,* 6, 18.

Sackett DL, Rosenberg WM, Gray JA, Haynes RB, Richardson WS (1996) Evidence-based medicine: what it is and what it isn't. *Br Med J,* 312, 71–72.

Schmidt HG, Norman GR, Boshuizen HPA (1990) A cognitive perspective on medical expertise: theory and implications. *Acad Med,* 65, 611–621.

Schön DA (1983) The Reflective Practitioner: How Professionals Think in Action. London: Temple Smith.

Shanafelt T, Dyrbye L (2012) Oncologist burnout: causes, consequences and responses. *J Clin Oncol,* 30, 1235–1241.

Silverman J, Kurtz S, Draper J (2005) *Skills for Communicating with Patients,* 2nd edition. Abingdon: Radcliffe Medical Press.

Sinclair S (1997) *Making Doctors: An Institutional Apprenticeship (Explorations in Anthropology).* Oxford: Berg 3PL.

Spurgeon P, Clark J, Ham C (2011) *Medical Leadership: From the Dark Side to the Centre Stage.* London: Radcliffe Publishing Ltd.

Stephan WG, Stephan CW (1996) Predicting prejudice. *Int J Inter Relat,* 20, 409–426.

Swanwick T, McKimm J (2014) Faculty development for leadership and management. In: Steinert Y (ed.), *Faculty Development in the Health Professions: A Focus on Research and Practice.* Dordrecht: Springer.

ten Cate O (2013) Nuts and bolts of entrustable professional activities. *J Grad Med Educ,* 5 (1), 157–158.

The American Nurses Association (ANA) (2001) *Code of Ethics for Nurses.* ANA.

The American Society of Consultant Pharmacists (ASCP) (2002) *Statement on Patient Advocacy*. ASCP.

The Royal College of Physicians and Surgeons of Canada (2005) *The CanMEDS Framework*. The Royal College of Physicians and Surgeons of Canada.

The Royal College of Psychiatrists (RCP) (2011) *Mental Health of Students in Higher Education*. London: RCP.

Thomas M, Burt M, Parkes J (2010) The emergence of evidence-based practice. In: McCarthy J, Rose P (eds.), *Values-Based Health and Social Care. Beyond Evidence-Based Practice*. London: Sage, pp. 3–24.

Thornton T (2006) Tacit knowledge as the unifying factor in evidence-based medicine and clinical judgment. *Philos Ethics Humanit Med*, 1, E2.

Till A, Pettifer G, O'Sullivan H, McKimm J (2014) Developing and harnessing the leadership potential of doctors in training. *Br J Hosp Med (Lond)*, 75 (9), 281–285.

Truong M, Paradies Y, Priest N (2014) Interventions to improve cultural competency in healthcare: a systematic review of reviews. *BMC Health Serv Res*, 14, 99. www.biomedcentral.com/1472-6963/14/99

Tuckman BW, Jenson MAC (1977) Stages of small group development revisited. *Group Organ Stud*, 2, 419–427.

UK Central Council for Nursing, Midwifery and Health Visiting (UKCC) (1992) *The Code of Professional Conduct*. UKCC.

University of Sydney (2012) *Academic Dishonesty and Plagiarism in Coursework Policy*. http://sydney.edu.au/arts/downloads/documents/policy/academic_dishonesty_in_coursework_policy_2012.pdf

Van de Ridder JMM, Stokking KM, McGaghie WC, ten Cate OTJ (2008) What is feedback in clinical education? *Med Educ*, 42, 189–197.

Vogan CL, McKimm J, Da Silva A, Grant AJ (2014) Twelve tips for providing effective student support in undergraduate medical education. *Med Teach*, 36 (6), 480–485.

Williams R (1999) Cultural safety – what does it mean for our work practice? *Aust N Z J Public Health*, 23 (2), 213–214.

Wright E, Holcombe C, Salmon P (2004) Doctors' communication of trust, care and respect in breast cancer. *Br Med J*, 328, 864–870.

Wynia MK, Papdakis MA, Sullivan WM, Hafferty FW (2014) More than just a list of values and desired behaviours: a foundational understanding of medical professionalism. *Acad Med*, 89, 712–714.

# Further reading

## Part 1: Professionalism in context

Irvine D, Johnson N, Thistlethwaite J, Hundt GL (2010) Professionalism: the UK perspective. In: D Bhugra, A Malik (eds.), *Professionalism in Mental Healthcare: Experts, Expertise and Expectations*. Cambridge: Cambridge University Press, pp. 48–61.

A summary of historical factors leading to a reconceptualization of professionalism in the UK. The lead author is a former president of the General Medical Council.

Foucault, M (1963) *The birth of the clinic: an archeology of medical perception*. New York: Routledge

Freidson, E (2006) *Professional dominance: the social dominance of medical care*. New York: Atherton Press.

Thistlethwaite JE, Spencer J (2008) *Professionalism in Medicine*. Oxford: Radcliffe Medical Press.

Expands on many of the topics in this book – useful for medical students, doctors in training and teachers.

Porter R (1997) *The Greatest Benefit to Mankind. A Medical History of Humanity from Antiquity to the Present Day*. London: Harper Collins.

## Part 2: Learning to be a professional
### Medical Education

Swanwick T (ed.) (2014) *Understanding Medical Education: Evidence, Theory and Practice*, 2nd edition. Chichester: Wiley-Blackwell/ASME.

A comprehensive book covering many aspects of medical education including learning and teaching, assessment, selection and remediation.

### Assessment

Davis M, McKimm J, Forrest K (2013) *How to Assess Doctors and Health Professionals*. Chichester: Wiley-Blackwell/BMJ Books.

Varian F, Cartwright L (2013) *The Situational Judgement Test at a Glance*. Chichester: Wiley-Blackwell.

### Plagiarism

www.ithenticate.com/plagiarism-detection-blog

iThenticate is a software programme for detecting plagiarism used by many journals. The webpages have examples of common problems and lists the top 10 plagiarism scandals of each year.

## Part 3: Professionalism in practice

McKimm J, Forrest K (2011) *Professional Practice for Foundation Doctors*. Exeter: Learning Matters Ltd.

### Emotional intelligence and emotional labour

Goleman D (1996) *Emotional Intelligence: Why It Can Matter More Than IQ*. New York, NY: Bantam Doubleday Dell Publishing Group.

Hochschild AR (2012) *The Managed Heart: Commercialization of Human Feeling*. Berkley: University of California Press.

Kasman D, Fryer-Edwards K, Braddock C (2003) Educating for professionalism: trainees' emotional experiences on IM and pediatrics inpatient wards. *Acad Med*, 78, 730–741.

Shoenberg P, Yakeley J (eds.) (2014) *Learning about Emotions in Illness*. Hove: Routledge.

### Reflective practice

Grant A (2005) *Reflection and Medical Students' Learning*. Saarbrüchen: Lambert Academic Publishing.

### Ethics

http://bma.org.uk/ethics

Useful resources covering ethics for students and practical advice.

### Evidence-based practice

Glasziou P, del Mar C, Salisbury J (2007) *Evidence-Based Practice Workbook*, 2nd edition. London: BMJ Books.

Heneghan C, Badenoch D (2006) *Evidence-Based Medicine Toolkit*, 2nd edition. London: BMJ Books.

### Practical guides

Goldacre B (2009) *Bad Science*. London: Fourth Estate.

How data are manipulated and distorted in the name of science and evidence. Entertaining and stimulating.

### Values-based practice

Seedhouse D (2005) *Values-Based Decision Making for the Caring Professions*. Chichester: John Wiley & Sons.

### Cultural competency

www.acog.org/Resources-And-Publications/Committee-Opinions/Committee-on-Health-Care-for-Underserved-Women/Cultural-Sensitivity-and-Awareness-in-the-Delivery-of-Health-Care

American College of Obstetrics and Gynaecology: set of useful resources on cultural competency and awareness in the delivery of healthcare with case study examples.

## Part 4: Working with patients
### Communication and shared decision-making

Hoffmann TC, Légaré F, Simmons MB, McNamara K, McCaffery K, Trevena LJ, Hudson B, Glasziou PP, Del Mar CB (2014) Shared decision making: what do clinicians need to know and why should they bother? *Med J Aust*, 201(1), 35–39.

Thistlethwaite JE (2005) Patient partnership and shared decision making: involving patients in management decisions. *Health Issues*, 83, 22–25.

### Useful review articles
### *Quality improvement*

The Health Foundation (2013) *Quality Improvement Made Simple*. London: The Health Foundation.

### *Patient portals*

www.healthit.gov/providers-professionals/faqs/what-patient-portal

US-based website explaining what portals are with useful links.

## Part 5: Working with others

**Teamwork and collaborative practice**

Hammick M, Freeth D, Copperman J, Goodsman D (2009) *Being Interprofessional*. Cambridge: Polity.

Reeves S, Lewin S, Espin S, Zwarenstein M (2010) *Interprofessional Teamwork for Health and Social Care*. London: Blackwell.

For more in depth reading – research and discussion about models of care and evaluation of these.

Panesar, SS, Carson-Stevens, A, Salvilla, SA, Sheikh, A (2014) *Patient safety and healthcare improvement at a glance,* Chichester, Wiley-Blackwell

Thistlethwaite JE (2012) *Values-Based Interprofessional Collaborative Practice*. Cambridge: Cambridge University Press.

For health professionals, focussing on teams and working together with case histories.

World Health Organization (2010) *Framework for Action on Interprofessional Education and Collaborative Practice*. Geneva: WHO.

The rationale and research behind interprofessional education and team-based care.

**Leadership**

McKimm J, O'Sullivan H (2012–2014) *Br J Hospital Med.* Aspects of Leadership Series.

A series of articles covering a wide range of clinical leadership topics, many relevant to students and doctors in training.

Swanwick T, McKimm J (2011) *The ABC of Clinical Leadership.* Chichester: Wiley-Blackwell.

## Part 6: Professional issues and dilemmas

Monrouxe LV, Rees CE (2012) "It's just a clash of cultures": emotional talk within medical students' narratives of professionalism dilemmas. *Adv Health Sci Educ Theory Pract*, 17, 671–701.

Monrouxe LV, Rees CE, Endacott R, Ternan E (2014) 'Even now it makes me angry': health care students' professionalism dilemma narratives. *Med Educ*, 48, 502–517.

Rees CE, Monrouxe LV, McDonald LA (2013) Narrative, emotion and action: analysing 'most memorable' professionalism dilemmas. *Med Educ*, 47, 80–96.

# Index